VAGINAL POLITICS:
A Midwife's Story

Bluwaters Press

Presents

VAGINAL POLITICS:
A Midwife's Story

an

Oral History

by Judy Lee

as told to

Bette Waters

VAGINAL POLITICS:
A Midwife's Story

Lee, Judy, 1946-
    Vaginal Politics: a midwife's story: an oral history
/by Judy Lee; as told to Bette Waters.
    p.cm.
    At head of title: Bluwaters Press Presents
    Includes bibliographical references.
    ISBN 09665584-7-2

    1. Lee, Judy, 1946- 2. Midwives--United States--
Biography.   I. Waters, Bette L. II. Title.
    III. Title. At head of title: Bluwaters Press presents

    RG950.L435A3 2003   618.2'0092
                                   QBI03-2003394

        Editors Ann Sallemi and Margaret Loring

        Cover Design JacDonald Jones

        Cover Art Dorinda Beaumont,
                New York City

            10 9 8 7 6 5 4 3 2 1

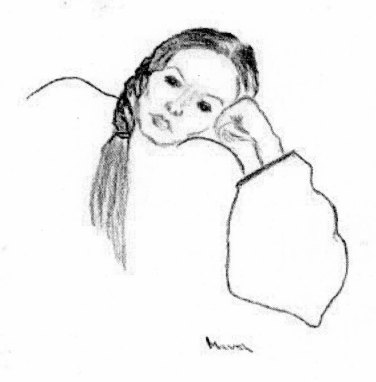

Judy Lee

by Marsh Brill - 1975

Bluwaters Press
P O Box 878
Mesilla, NM 88046

Other Publications by Bluwaters Press

Massage During Pregnancy, Third Edition
by Bette Waters 2004

Wayfayers: The Spiritual Journeys of Nicholas & Helena Roerich,
by Ruth Abrams Drayer 2004

High Seas Passage
by Billy A. McClellan 2004

Healing the Great White Lie
by Bette Waters 2004

One Foot Away From A Million
by Donald E. McCoy 2003

My Daddy Brought Me Up To Be Good
by Bette Waters 1999

Judy Lee

Contents

Judy Lee

Acknowledgements

The writing of this book has been my way of dealing with old issues. It has been a cleansing and healing process. My greatest wish for this biography is that it be used as a reminder that the world has changed because there were women out there on the frontier who were willing to fight the system to obtain and preserve their rights as patients.

It has given me the opportunity of looking back on a period that was very fretful and negative for me at the time. I never saw myself as being an incredibly strong person for having lived through it, until actually getting this down on paper. I had no awareness at the time of how much I was doing. My purpose as a midwife was to be a servant to women, one on one. I had no idea what the obtaining of the education to meet my goal, and later the living of the attainment of it, was going to require of me. I certainly did not view it as something needing anything unusual, or doing anything unusual. I was only doing what was necessary at the time.

People come into a life for a season or a reason or a lifetime. Here are some of my people.

Christmas Leubrie was the woman who told me about the direct entry route for midwifery education rather than nursing. She taught me the true meaning of radical feminism in action. Ira Director, drove me to midwifery school, in more ways than one; Max Marcus, MSW, author, counselor, guru, shaman, and dear friend to many; Karen Lux Michel for her been there, done that, bought the tee-shirt "friendship" and sustenance since kindergarten.

Marsh Brill, who is a perfect role model for all that is truly wild, wonderful and magical in a friendship. Marty, Romana and Dave (my brothers and sister) whose feedback is always on target and so loving. They sometimes make me cry before I crack up with laughter. A thank you to Patti Jo Dorsey who taught me in fifth grade that being a girl does not mean being a wimp; Patrick Brady, my boyfriend since fifth grade at St. Leo.

For Aunt Dorothy Marsh who taught me at least one different viewpoint at every turn of my life that helped me make courageous decisions.

For Jacquelyn D. Lee, my mother, John E. Lee, my daddy; Jay, my beloved son and Roberta, my dear daughter-in-law, for being part of the hope for a loving, creative and joy-filled future.

JUDY LEE
June 2003

Books do not get made alone. Don Williamson, retired English educator, always responds cheerfuly and promptly to my requests for help with grammar and punctuation expertise. John Arnold, who was educated by the Nuns, continues to teach me more about commas than I ever wanted to know. Working with Judy Lee has been one of the most *fun* things I have done this year. Ann Sallemi and Ruth Drayer continue to head the list of support persons I feel I can call upon for many things, from checking my Spanish to furnishing emotional support.

BETTE WATERS
June 2003

INTRODUCTION

By Bette Waters

The Writers' Group

As I grow older I am surprised when I am reminded of my age by the knowledge that many of the things that I take for granted are completely unknown to my children, grandchildren and their peers. But when I find that an institution where I am employed has conveniently forgotten its controversial history, I am beset with the desire to tell it to the world.

In the early 1980's I was a staff midwife at a hospital on the west coast of Florida. My curiosity was tweaked by the passing remark of a researcher about the hospital's history of placing laboring pregnant women in beds, giving them drugs to cause amnesia and tying nets over the beds so that the drugged women could not get out of bed. By the time the drug had worn off, she had had her baby and had no memory of what happened. This was one of the biggest reasons families were forbidden to accompany their laboring wives, daughters, etc. into the hospital labor rooms. If family members had witnessed how hard and violently the women struggled during each contraction under the influence of this drug, the medical profession would have been forced to handle laboring women differently. So, I wrote the book, *Healing the Great White Lie.*

The second event that touched me in this way was finding out that the hospital for which I was working as a staff midwife had been picketed by pregnant mothers in 1982. The physicians on staff were accused of refusing emergency care to patients of a midwife.

Young women graduating today from direct entry midwife schools and nurse-midwife education programs find it difficult to imagine what midwives experienced in the pioneering of the practice of midwifery in the United States in the 1970's and 80's. It is hard to believe that just 30 years ago, the mainstream medical profession looked upon women who wished to offer midwifery services to the public as being almost as evil as the midwives and witches of the early days of Salem.

During these years, attempts by the male-dominated medical profession to suppress women who were midwives was done with all the zeal used in their previous active take-over of the health and healing business, a take-over that had been supported and achieved within the institutions and political realms of our society.[1]

And so it was to these political institutions that midwives, attempting to gain acceptance and the legal right to their professional roles in our health care system, took their battle. The state and federal laws were challenged in the courts and on the floor of state legislators. No easy task, but over long years the professional midwives won.[2] But at what price?

The price was exacted not only from the midwives seeking to care for mothers and babies, but from the mothers and babies themselves. Women who had been frightened out of their homes to give birth in hospitals under the guise of safety, found the hospital procedures and standards traumatized them both physically and emotionally. Furthermore, the women were sold a bill of goods that said, "a good mother is willing to sacrifice anything for her baby." Then she was sent home to stuff her pain and cope alone.

Allopathic medicine treated women and babies in the hospital setting in such a way that, in 1986, Dr. Thomas Brewer, a leading expert on metabolic toxicity of pregnancy observed, "A child[3] in a neonatal intensive care unit is an abused child." As a result of the patients' rights movement that began in the 1960's women began to assert themselves by choosing home births and birthing centers with midwives. Allopathic medicine went to great lengths to protect their turf against these professional midwives.

---

1. Ehrenreich, B. English, D. *Witches, Midwives, and Nurses: A History of Women Healers.* Feminist Press at The City University of New York, New York, NY. 1973.

2. Suarez, S. H. *Midwifery Is Not The Practice of Medicine.* Yale Journal of Law and Feminism, Vol. 5(2), Spring 1993.

3. Brewer, T., MD. Address at NAPSAC Summit, 1986.

This is a story of one of these women, Judy Lee, professional midwife who was harassed by local physicians in legal and illegal arenas. It is a story of professional and personal sacrifice. It is a story of a brave and courageous woman who worked long hours to help women. It is the story of emotional trauma buried within her psyche. This emotional trauma when tapped 25 years later, resembled the trauma suppression seen in women who have been violently raped and never told anyone about it.

I met Judy Lee in 1999 at a weekend seminar at my church. We were assigned to the same small work group for two days. The group talked about near and dear issues and our personal spirituality. Judy and I hit it off immediately. I liked how she presented herself, and her warmth put me at ease. After the seminar, we continued to have lunches discussing books, movies and other interests. It was not until several weeks later that we learned that we were both midwives.

Judy was no longer working as a midwife. She had recently moved back to Las Cruces after living for many years in California. We both rejoiced in finding this new connection but I do not remember that we talked much about our different work experiences. It seemed that our friendship encompassed so many other things than work stuff.

In 1997, I semi-retired from my job as staff midwife at the local hospital and began devoting more of my time to writing. I was a published author of a book written for the Massage Therapy profession, *Massage During Pregnancy*. Also, I had kept a journal for the previous 30 years and had written poetry. However, I longed to be part of a writing community. After looking around and checking out my acquaintances, I decided that the only way I was going to become part of a writing community was to start my own group.

Our writing group was made up of two other midwives, a semi-retired significant other, a retired former dance teacher and pianist, myself and our newest member, Judy Lee. Our meeting format had each member read aloud from her writings, and then receive critique from the others while we all munched snacks.

It was Judy's turn to read. She began. A short way into the first page, tears began running down her cheeks and she struggled to control her voice. One of the midwife members of the group gently took the papers from her hand and continued the story, reading for her.

"It was a professional job and an expensive one at that. They are getting better at it. We found the equipment up a phone pole about a mile down the road," the detective scowled.

"What kind of pervert would want to record my conversations about the color of blood and intensity of pain?" she asked in bewilderment. "And how does this tie in with the obscene phone calls and death threats?"

Although he had decided months ago that he genuinely liked this woman, he was still irritated at her naivete. "Now think about it! You used to be a big city girl," he growled, spraying his words like an Uzi. "Who has plenty of money? Who could easily pay to have this done? Who would want to get something, anything, on you? Who has the most to gain by scaring you out of the midwife business?"

Suddenly honeysuckle enveloping the porch made the spring night air sickeningly sweet. Her knees buckled as she reached for the arm of the swing to sit down. Barely audible was the "Oh" she gasped as the seriousness of the situation finally began to dawn on her.

Seeing her tremble, Martin tempered his tone and spoke more gently. "This isn't a game, Judy. This is the third time we've found their wiretaps. You must realize that they mean business and they know who you are and where you live. This isn't just you and your little pregnant migrant workers anymore. You are hitting them in their wallet and they have already shown that they will do anything to protect their livelihood. And more importantly, their egos. They must discredit you publicly and run you out of town."

She did not hear much more of what he said. She was mostly numb and deaf sitting there shivering despite the southwest heat. She sat on the porch for a long time after he pulled away—looking over the chile fields but not really seeing them or the mountains beyond, despite the bright glow of the al-

most-full moon.

Lying in bed later, still awake as the sun rose, over and over again she kept thinking, I have got to answer the phone and open the door in the middle of the night. My women are counting on me.

During lunch the next day Judy, shared with me the great surprise she had the night before our writers' meeting. In bed, propped among great pillows with her yellow legal pad, trying to think of something meaningful to write about, she thought about being a midwife. Maybe a birth story would be the place to begin.

Shortly, with pen to paper, the words began to flow along with a flood of tears. She had written only half a page and looked down at the tear-stained paper almost as though she was transported back to a time when she had been too exhausted to allow herself to feel. She told me how shocked and upset she was upon discovering her visceral reaction to the memories.

In the following months, she would tell me pieces of events during those years. Although she had been forced by her sense of self-preservation to walk away from it, the pain had been stiffled and she was expending a tremendous amount of energy keeping the feelings down.

I am a ravenous reader and love spending time in second-hand bookstores. Browsing, touching, scanning book covers is like therapy for me, soothing, reassuring, relaxing. I was in one of the world's best used bookstores, COAS My Bookstore, Las Cruces, New Mexico, when I found a book entitled, *Like It Was,* by Cynthia Stokes Brown. It was a complete guide to writing oral histories. I was fascinated by the idea of oral histories. I had been writing oral medical histories in patients' charts for twenty-plus years. Over the years I have experienced receiving a book intended for a specific purpose. I knew this was that kind of book when I began to read it.

I wanted to write a book about Judy's experience as a midwife using the oral history format. I approached Judy with the idea and she was interested. But she was not sure she could bring herself to dredge up all the memories. We talked about it and she began to understand that if she had that kind of visceral reaction recalling just a small portion, it was material that needed to see the light of day. And so it was decided.

Judy felt that talking into a tape recorder would be acceptable, since we could do it at her home, a place where she felt safe. In the living room of Judy's lovely adobe, surrounded with energy created in this space, lavish with art and sculpture and three loving dogs, we began.

The first session started without much preplanning or decisions about any particular order of the material. We decided to just let it flow freely. Judy was comfortable with the microphone clipped to her blouse and we proceeded as though we were having one of our friendly fun conversations, giggling over hiding the recorder and allowing the dogs to choose their favorite spots.

She had been talking for about half an hour when she began to feel the fear and anxiety rise to the surface. Her shaking and trembling returned and the tears began to fall. We took a break for her to perform some deep breathing and receive a few encouraging licks from the dogs, who sensed her anxiety. Then she was ready to continue.

We had four more recording sessions over the next few months. These sessions were planned to fill in gaps and were guided with my questions. The final number of recorded hours was approximately eight. Judy was able to move through these sessions with only small twinges from time to time.

During the years she operated her midwifery service, she was involved in events that were considered newsworthy at the time. She had saved many newspaper clippings outlining the sequence of events and the controversy her practice created among local physicians and within the community. She recalled that articles appeared in newspapers as far away as Arizona, Colorado and Texas, as well as New Mexico.

Some of these newspapers clippings from the *El Paso Times* in El Paso, Texas, did not have dates on them. I wrote to the archive librarian at the Times and received permission to research these dates in their library.

Judy accompanied me to this appointment. To our great surprise, when we introduced ourselves to the librarian, she handed us two large worn, brown manila envelopes labeled "Judy Lee". Now we knew that Judy Lee was famous and perhaps even infamous. We sat for several hours pouring over the clippings. Many Judy did not have in her files. The librarian was friendly and made copies of all the stories for us. Many of these rich files appear as part of this book.

This is her story and the story of her well-loved and courageous "pregos".

JUDY'S STORY
As Told To Bette Waters

Part I

The Process

The Community

In 1979 when I graduated from The Maternity Center in El Paso, Texas, I really wanted to work with Hispanic migrant women. I scoped out the rural areas around El Paso. Anthony was half way between Las Cruces, New Mexico, and El Paso, and infact, straddled the border, with part of the town in each state. The nearest hospitals were located in either Las Cruces or El Paso. There were only two doctors in Anthony at the time. Both were general practitioners and did not do any kind of prenatal care or deliveries.

I decided I would look for office space in Anthony. I went around and introduced myself to Mayor Adrian Baca. He was really happy with the idea of having me move into the community. He introduced me to the two pharmacists in town, Fernando Palafox, and Danny Sanchez and a few other people. He told them with great gusto that I would be coming to town and asked that they support me.

The mayor actually helped me find a place to rent that was suitable for a birthing center. He showed me a mother-in-law type house behind a house. So, I set up my first birth center in Anthony, Texas, on Third Street south of Franklin, behind the La Feria grocery store.

The building needed lots of repairs. I had to put up ceilings and walls. The electricity had not been used in years. I ran new wires to the building and had an electrician come in and wire a box. I dug a 30-foot trench with a pick ax through the super-hard caliche across the back yard to the other house to hook into the gas line.

The women in the town began showing up before I was finished with the renovations. I would put down the pick ax, or climb down the ladder, or wipe plaster off my hands, or prop the new drywall in a convenient place, then talk to them.

I felt the place was beautiful. I had a big living room for my Lamaze classes. It was a really great facility and the house was in Texas. I was still only licensed in Texas, actually only in the county of El Paso, because the State of Texas did not have licensing. I had to keep my physical practice on the Texas side.

Most of the back yard was in New Mexico. The laboring women really liked being in the back yard under the trees. I jokingly told them they could walk around; but if they decided to have the baby out there, they had to return beyond a particular tree in the yard so they would be in Texas. That would keep me out of trouble for delivering a baby in New Mexico.

Although I had no license to practice in New Mexico, the state would issue me a license if I sat for their exam and passed. My educational credentials and my experience, demonstrated by the high number of deliveries done as a student, qualified me to take and pass the New Mexico exam. However, they had not offered the exam in something like twenty years. Back then, New Mexico had "granny midwives" and "parteras". They were doing home deliveries without a license. But I was fearful of practicing without a license.

During the start-up of my practice, I had a partner. Georgette D'Amour was a nurse and a midwife with whom I had gone to school in El Paso. She was from California. After I opened my birth center, she moved back here to be a midwife with me.

Her mother was elderly and Georgette was responsible for supporting her. We were working primarily with an indigent population and were getting paid a lot in chickens, onions, chile, or people doing laundry or yard work. Unfortunately, Georgette was not licensed to practice nursing in Texas or New Mexico. Otherwise, she could have supplemented her income. In a very short time she decided to move back to California. Then I was practicing alone.

Anthony Times   **March 1979**

Birthways Opens In Anthony

Two midwives, legally registered by the State of Texas, are providing full prenatal care, Lamaze type childbirth prepa-

rations classes and home delivery services here in Anthony. Judy Lee and Georgette D'Amour have founded Birthways to offer personal, family centered care to those healthy women who are choosing home birth. Classes and services are offered in English and Spanish. Birthways is located directly behind the new shopping center at 301 South Third Street.

The former dentist's office has been renovated and redesigned to meet the needs of the birthing women and her family. Ms. Lee says, "We expect to be attending about 10 births a month. About half of these will deliver in their own homes, with those women living outside Texas delivering in our lovely new Birthing Room here."

Ms. Lee is originally from Chicago and has been practicing midwifery in the El Paso area for over a year. Ms. D'Amour is a registered nurse and midwife who has recently arrived from the San Francisco Bay area. While working together in 1977, Lee and D'Amour conceived the idea of Birthways. Both women believe pregnancy is a normal, healthy function of a woman's body. Prenatal care and delivery services are viewed as a very important part of an entire health continuum. They believe that midwives and other professionals must coordinate their areas of expertise to best serve their clients. Birthways clients are encouraged to work with local M.D.s, nurse practitioners, chiropractors, counselors, etc., in order to develop a full range of health care programs for their families.

"The pregnant woman is much more complex and important than her medical charts reflect," says Ms. Lee.

An Holistic attitude is maintained while dealing with each woman as a total person. Ms. D'Amour has her Master's Degree in Public Health and 13 years experience in this field. She is convinced, "Each client must be viewed as part of their own larger environment in order to be cared for most effectively. Particular attention to the family unit and extended family situations is essential. The special needs of first-time mothers and single-parent families must also be addressed.

"Birthways maintains a position of non-interference; while physician consultation, laboratory tests and the best technologies are used continually to screen for safety. A new national concept in health promotion and education has been piloted by Birthways with the introduction of their Mobile Unit." This emergency transport vehicle will serve the dual purpose of providing full-range health screening services to isolated areas of the community.

Both Judy and Georgette provide all prenatal services in order to become personally and well acquainted with each client before the delivery. Fathers are encouraged to participate in all phases of care to prepare them for the option of coaching and "catching" at the birth of their child. The midwives are also providing free lectures and slide show presentations on a variety of related subjects to schools, women's organizations and community groups. Family planning, home birth, new baby care, and breast feeding are some of the topics they explore.

The migrant workers did not care where they delivered. My birthing center was fine for them. In fact, many of them told me over and over again how thrilled they were to have their baby born "in such a beautiful home".

Although it was small, it was cheerful and it was nice to hear that they appreciated my efforts. Soon I started getting middle class women from New Mexico. They wanted home births. I could not do the home births because I had no New Mexico license. Some women offered me two or three hundred dollars extra and "promised not to tell". My conscience would not let me do that. It was not a safety issue being across the street from the New Mexico, Texas state line. It was a professional issue. I knew that I would risk losing my license it if I did that. I also had my son to think about.

Also, people approached me wanting to buy birth certificates for babies. They offered me two to three thousand dollars cash so their kids could be US citizens. I never dreamed that sort of thing existed. And of course, I refused.

I made arrangements with the ambulance company to park their ambulance outside my birthing center. The drivers would sit in my waiting room and drink coffee during births. This allowed a transfer to the hospital in fifteen minutes if I had a problem.

Many of my patients were residents of Texas, but soon I was doing a lot of births for New Mexico women. My New Mexico mothers did not want to be transferred to Texas if there was a problem, so I went to see the owner of the ambulance company in Las Cruces. I set it up so that when I had a New Mexico woman delivering at my birthing center, they would come down and park in front. They could leave if they had another call. They charged me $25, the same fee that they charged the automobile drag race track to park their ambulance at the track during races. If there was a problem, they would be there. I built that into my fees. I paid directly each time they came. If they transported a patient, they charged for the transport and the woman would be responsible for the fee. I had almost no transports, but having an ambulance right there made me feel much better.

In the long, run this attempt to increase safety for my patients pulled me into the politics of health care in ways I would never have considered under different circumstances. Texas, as well as New Mexico, had Emergency Medical Technicians (EMT), as opposed to paramedics staffing the ambulance systems. This was a real issue for me. I wanted the increased safety of paramedics on the ambulances; their scope of practice is significantly wider than that of an EMT. One of the main things that concerned me was EMT's could not set up an IV or give any drugs. I had been trained to set up an IV, but legally I could not do so.

Even in my first year in practice, I had very few transports, but I wanted to be ready for anything. Within the first six months of practice, my fears played out. I delivered this woman and the delivery went fine. The placenta showed the typical signs of separation, but it would not come out. It did not come and it did not come. Suddenly she started dumping huge amounts of blood. I went in to perform a manual removal of the placenta. The placenta had peeled off, but over to one side I found a silver dollar size piece of placenta that had actually grown through the wall of the uterus. The medical term for this is Placenta Accreta, a rare occurrence.

I removed the rest of the placenta and performed external bimanual compression, squeezing from the outside to keep the uterus clamped down to decrease the bleeding. I had a standing order from a physician to administer Pitocin (a drug that causes the uterus to contract and decreases bleeding) in such emergencies. I gave it to her intramuscularly. We wasted no time loading mother and baby into the ambulance that was parked just outside.

During the transport, the EMT's called in to the hospital in El Paso three different times, telling the staff in the emergency room this was not a retained placenta, it was true Placenta Accreta. I gave them her blood type so that they could start a cross match and asked them to be ready for us with the surgery suite and surgeon ready. I told them she was going to need either a hysterectomy or some kind of surgical intervention. The ambulance people even let me talk to the hospital on the radio because I was sure by their responses they were not understanding the urgency.

EMT's could not set up an IV or even MAST pants (pneumatic anti-shock trousers) so I asked them for tourniquets. I put one on each of her legs and one on her arm and I moved it to the other arm half way through the transport.

Sure enough, when we arrived at the hospital, they were not ready for us, nor was an obstetrician in the emergency room waiting for us. I had to stand there and wait covered with blood. They had way more nursing staff and people in the emergency room than you would normally see. They were all nosing about, looking to see what was going on. They were laughing that I was trying to stop a uterine hemorrhage by putting tourniquets on her arms and legs.

The doctor came in and examined her. His response was "Holy shit, it is accreta. In 20 years of practice, I've never seen one." They whisked her off to the surgery suite. Nobody offered me a place to sit down, a cup of coffee or anything. They just kept walking past looking at me all bloody. Finally, one nurse came over to where I was leaning against the wall and offered me a pair of scrubs and a wash cloth and told me I could go in their bathroom and get cleaned up. I felt so touched by her compassion.

I was still worried about my poor woman. The doctor who came down to do the exam turned out to be the head of the OB department. After the surgery, he returned to the ER.

He called me and everybody else—there had to be a good 10 to 15 people—into this private room in the ER. In a mean voice, he said, "I want to talk to you young lady!"

I was waiting to get grilled. The nurses were all tee-heeing and talking to each other because I was going to get into trouble. "Were you trying to stop a uterine hemorrhage by putting tourniquets on her arms and legs?" he asked.

"No sir," I replied, "I wasn't. I was just trying to keep the blood in her body core to give her brain and heart as much oxygen as possible."

He turned to the nurses, asking, "Would any of you have had enough common sense to do that?" He dismissed them. He walked over and put his arm around me and said, "You used really good judgment and I would be proud to help you out and see your patients. I will help you any way that I can."

I decided to use him as a back up physician. And he kept to his word. Once I got licensed in New Mexico, state regulations for midwives required that every patient I planned to deliver have two visits with a physician: one exam early in the pregnancy where she would have labs reviewed and the second visit after the end of her 36th week. He let my women make partial payments even on their two visits.

After that, I had a few non-emergency transports to that hospital, but they were mostly women getting dehydrated or exhausted and needing a little glucose. We would take them in the ambulance to the hospital. Once they got an IV, their energy level returned and they could deliver their babies normally.

This doctor instructed the nurses to let him know when my patients were ready to be taken to the delivery suite. He would come to the labor room and send the nurses off to do errands. Then he would stand there saying things like, "Oh, Judy, I'm having a hard time getting my gloves on, so why don't you just catch this one."

He never cut an episiotomy and we never took any of them to the delivery room. I don't know that he would want anybody to know that. He is still practicing. He was a really great supporter.

At that time, there were no EMT classes in this part of New Mexico. I wanted to be an EMT and a paramedic. I talked to the New Mexico Health Department in Santa Fe, the state capital, concerning the location of their training classes. The only place one could get certified as an EMT in New Mexico was in Albuquerque, 240 miles north of Las Cruces.

There were two rural migrant community heath centers in our area that were funded at the Federal level to provide health care for the poor. La Clinica de Familia in San Miguel, and Ben Archer located in the little town of Hatch, 45 miles north of Las Cruces. Ben Archer agreed to sponsor EMT classes if I could get Santa Fe to send someone to to teach the classes. Later, as part of the outreach program to improve services in the southern part of the state, we got our wish. Classes included the introduction of a permanent EMT training program at the Dona Ana Branch Community College in Las Cruces.

I enrolled in the very first class held at the Ben Archer Health Center. It was so much fun. The classes were taught on Saturday and Sunday from eight o'clock in the morning until three in the afternoon. On Friday night, I would drive up to Elephant Butte Lake. To save money, I camped in a tent. Then I drove to the Ben Archer Clinic on Saturday morning. I had my beeper with me in case anyone went into labor.

Through all those weeks and weeks of classes nobody went into labor until after three p.m. on Sunday. It was like a miracle.

In the past, when I had gone camping, I would never once make it through a whole weekend without getting called back for a birth. I felt it was some kind of sign that getting this training was exactly the correct thing. There was no opportunity to make up for missed classes and I would not have completed the course.

For some reason, the doctors at the hospital did not want paramedics. Privately, I went to the head doctor of the emergency room. He was the one having to deal with all the sick and injured coming in. The emergency room doctor had no problem with having paramedics. He had worked with them in other places. The level of care necessary when people were transported by paramedics was much less problematic than if they had been initially treated by EMT's.

These were two big issues for me, paramedics on the ambulance and prenatal care for the indigent. I worked with the emergency room doctor and the new group at Dona Ana Branch in an attempt to get Santa Fe to approve a paramedic class in Dona Ana County. I also attended the first paramedic class in Las Cruces.

The paramedics class was headed up by a wonderful woman, Patti Silver. She inspired everyone she touched. She moved the program forward at a fast pace, kept the students on task and was very professional.

We also had fun. Nobody wanted me for a partner to practice setting up IV's because my veins were small and rolled badly. I could not pass that module without a partner. Patti solved my partner problem. She realized why no one wanted to try on me. She offered credit for three IV setups to anyone who successfully started an IV on my veins!

I was teaching emergency childbirth to the medical technicians. After certification as a paramedic, I began teaching the paramedics emergency childbirth at the university. All of the paramedics and the people who worked on the ambulance system had been my students or my classmates. It was a wonderful set up.

I extended my emergency childbirth class to the fire departments around Las Cruces and Anthony and a lot of the volunteer fire departments out in the county. You could not have had a better captive audience. These guys were terrified at the thought of having to deliver a baby. They were great students. They paid rapt attention to everything I said. Later, I was invited to teach this course for the police department and the sheriff's office.

I received a two year appointment to work with a group at New Mexico State University. The main focus of the program was to determine what needed to be taught in schools. What kind of sex education should we be doing? There was no sex education at all happening in the schools in New Mexico at that time.

Despite not being approved by the State of New Mexico, I was invited several times to Gadsen High School to talk about sex education to their students because they had such a high teen pregnancy rate. I do not know how they circumvented the county school administration. The parents were asked to sign a permit for their children to attend my class, which consisted mostly of juniors and seniors.

I would teach them how to put condoms on bananas while dealing with all the tittering that teenagers go through. I had the wildest questions from those classes. If you douche with coca cola, can you still get pregnant? If you do it standing up, can you still get pregnant?

My response was, "First of all, let me congratulate you on your agility if you can do it standing up. Yes, you can still get pregnant."

I was invited by the Nursing School and the School of Sociology at New Mexico State University in Las Cruces to be a guest speaker. There was a lot of talk around the campus by the nursing students about my lecture. When I actually showed up to talk, the classroom they had originally planned to use was much too small. They took a short break and moved us to a bigger auditorium.

After the first lecture, one of the organizers came up to me and said that they had done a little headcount in the auditorium and found that there were way more faculty and students present than were actually enrolled in the nursing school.

We discussed such things as sex, self-pleasuring, lesbianism, gay love, how to prevent date rape, abortion, birth settings, and birth control options. The lectures were on-going and there was always a question and answer portion.

There had already been some publicity in the newspapers about doctors being upset with midwives, so the question period always included some inquiries about why doctors did not like midwives. I tried to be as tactful as possible, but when people continued to push me on the issue, I would explain that it was vaginal politics. It had to do with the male-controlled medical system keeping women in the appropriate setting, the hospitals, and continuing to making money on the birthing process.

I gave examples of male doctors withholding records from women and threatening to withhold birth control pills or any followup care after their babies were born if they decided to birth with a midwife.

Besides teaching seminars and having discussion groups at the university, I also worked with the local Right To Life group. They would send women to me for deliveries and help them pay for the pregnancy. We had a little closet for donated maternity clothes, cribs, buggies, high-chairs and carseats.

I also saw military wives. I really felt they needed to learn about pregnancy prevention and the side effects of using abortion as post-conception birth control. Abortions were very common practice on military bases. Most of the women had no idea about the side effects of scar tissue and the potential for creating problems with future pregnancies, as well as the possibility of puncturing the uterus.

The women were shocked that IUD's had potential side effects. Almost none of them knew that an IUD did not prevent conception, that it caused an early miscarriage by not allowing implantation in the uterine wall. Doctors who were passing out these devices at the time were not giving this kind of information or practicing true, informed consent.

Also, I assisted a few lesbian couples with information on artificial self-insemination while warning of the dangers of the newly discovered AIDS virus. Using their friends' semen and cervical caps or diaphragms, or even turkey basters on occasion, several of these women became pregnant and went on to be really great moms.

My teaching within the community was always joyful work. When I received feedback such as the following letter from Diana Lyon, a prison official, I felt that I truly did make a difference.

State of New Mexico
Corrections and Criminal Rehabilitation Department
Radium Springs Center For Women

Bruce King, Governor   Post Office Box 79
Roger Crist, Secretary   Radium Springs, NM 88054
Adolph Barela, Superintendent   (505)523-8531

December 4, 1981

Ms. Judy Lee
Route 1, Box 221
La Mesa, New Mexico 88044

Dear Judy:

This is a letter of support and commendation for the assistance you have provided residents of Radium Springs Center for Women as a professional midwife.

Your presentation on methods of family planning was explicit, concise and professional. You presented much needed information concerning the functioning of the female reproductive system. Incidentally many of our residents had no understanding of their bodies in spite of their street-wise upbringing. The film of an actual birth answered questions in a sensitive way for residents and staff alike.

So far, staff has not had to use the emergency childbirth training you presented. Knowing what emergency measures to take with our five (5) births has been invaluable. All concerned staff, other residents and the mothers were much calmer during transport to the delivery room.

Thank you for providing such sensitively presented

34

and practical prenatal service.

Sincerely,
Diana Lyon
Chief Classification Officer

During this time, I was bugging the health department to start a free prenatal care program for the indigent. They were not at all interested. The birth certificate clerical staff in Las Cruces turned into a strong ally in pressing for indigent prenatal care in the area.

Birth certificates were really important to the Hispanic population. I personally took my signed birth certificates to the county registrar in Las Cruces. It was my policy to hold off on filing the birth certificate until the mother had completed the three follow-up visits after her delivery. It was one way of forcing them to come back for their postpartum visits. I could have filed them immediately. Instead, I would just say that the birth certificate gets filled out after the two week check up. Once the baby was born, they had every thing they needed from me, they were not apt to follow up. Retaining the birth certificate was my way of making sure the baby was fine and that way I made sure the babies got their two week PKU tests performed.

Not only is a birth certificate proof of nationality and age, it also serves as a data collection tool, measuring local health care standards or lack thereof. One of the questions on the birth certificate is how many prenatal care visits did the mother have and starting at what month of the pregnancy. One day the registrar mentioned in passing that none of the hospital birth certificates provided that information. The hospital just left that item blank.

I certainly could not turn in a birth certificate with any portion left blank. Every space had to be filled out. I called Santa Fe to try to find out what the Bureau of Vital Statistics records showed. They hesitated once they realized they were talking to the midwife from Dona Ana County. They did not want to give me the information. I felt this had to be public information. I reminded them they were keeping vital statistics for the whole state. This information is required on birth certificates, and I wanted to know what our statistics were for Dona Ana County. Finally, they released the records.

The data for the particular month I was able to obtain showed 90 out of 100 births had no information available as to when or if prenatal care began. The report just read "not available, not available, not available." I recognized three of the births were babies that I delivered and I had given them the information.

The babies who were born at the hospital with documented prenatal care were anglo women who had paid obstetricians. I called the bureau in Santa Fe again and complained. If I had to fill out the birth certificates completely, then the doctors should have to fill them out completely.

The wheels of bureaucracy turn slowly, eventually they started to fill in these portions. The true answers of "unknown" or "no prenatal care" made for a much different picture than "not available". It turned out once the hospital started actually collecting that data from the nurses on the OB floor, something like 80% of women delivering there had no prenatal care. The outrageously high number of women with no prenatal care, combined with the press about me offering free prenatal care, put a lot of pressure on the health department.

During this time, Dr. Murray Bruder, Obstetrics and Gynecology practitioner in Las Cruces, who was President of the Dona Ana County Medical Association and Chief of Obstetrics at Memorial General Hospital, called the owner of the ambulance company. He told the owner that they should not be on call for any of my patients because it was dangerous. If they had a transport that was a stillbirth or if they had serious problems, they were going to get sued. Just by supporting the midwife, by being there, they were cooperating with something that was dangerous and illegal and immoral.

It was a small community and I knew the dispatcher for the ambulance company. Her husband was the coroner for the county. They were grand supporters of my practice and they told me about what Bruder had tried to do to the ambulance owner.

I had a very good relationship with the owner of the ambulance company who, over many months, had been hearing these wonderful stories. The owner told Bruder that it was good business and he was not going to be intimidated. If Bruder wanted to testify against the ambulance company if anything happened, he should go for it. But he was not backing down on doing backup for me.

If a woman was having her first baby, I would not call the ambulance until she was six or seven centimeters dilated. The paramedics stayed until after the placenta was delivered, the baby was stable and the newborn exam had been done.

I always made it a point to include the paramedics and EMT's in the birth as much as possible. As soon as the baby was born, the placenta was delivered and the cord was cut, I would ask the mother's permission to take the baby out into the living room so the paramedics could see it. The baby would still be slimy and slippery but wrapped in a warm towel. If the parents agreed, I let the women paramedics come into the bedroom and watch the birth.

It was the best marketing I could have ever done. The ambulance crews saw birth after birth after birth that were absolutely perfect. They knew we had few transports and that 95% of our transports were because the woman had become fatigued from laboring so long, or she was upset at her inability to handle the pain and would decide she wanted to be delivered at the hospital. This was rare, but I always honored the woman's decision.

The paramedics and the EMT's started having their own babies with me. Most of these people had insurance so it really helped subsidize all the free prenatal care I was doing.

A lot was going on at this time. I had passed the New Mexico exam for Licensed Midwife and this increased the number of patients from New Mexico.

In the Anthony area, there were many older people, men and women, under the care of doctors in El Paso. Their problems needing follow-up ranged from blood pressure checks, to need for iron injections or B12 shots. Once the doctors knew I was in Anthony and could give shots, they began to call me asking if I could go over and give Mrs. So-and-So her B12 shot. Or would I go over and take Mr. So-and-So's blood pressure and call it in.

I was sort of like the community's unofficial *enfermera*. It was fun. The doctors were prescribing the iron and giving me a standing order to administer it. The patients had the iron and needles at their homes. One lady always said when I gave her the shots, it never hurt, which was her way of showing gratitude. It was a real nice sense of community. There was one fellow who, by the time he was driven to the doctor's office and waited for his appointment, had pressure way up. If I took it at his house, then it was normal.

I remember going to an old man's house to take his blood pressure for his doctor in El Paso. He was sitting shirtless at the kitchen table with his wife. I could see the typical rash of shingles across his chest and back. He was miserable. He did not want me to put the blood pressure cuff on him.

One of the things I learned using natural remedies was how effective L-Lysine was for herpes. If my women with herpes took this every day, they never had an outbreak. So they did not have to have cesarean section delivery due to a current outbreak of herpes.

I went to my car and got my L-Lysine. Herpes is viral and so is shingles. I asked if he wanted to try it. He agreed, I suppose because he was in so much pain. I poured out my whole bottle of L-Lysine. We crushed about 10 pills and put them into hot water to melt and then added warm water. I dipped gauze in the mixture and placed it on his shingles covered skin. He experienced immediate relief. He started taking the L-Lysine orally. His wife continued with the applications. In less than a week, he was completely clear.

Back in those days, beepers were just becoming available, but I could not afford one. I was so poor I could not afford to buy an answering machine. One of the companies—a really sweet guy in El Paso—let me make monthly payments of $5 on both a beeper and answering machine.

Driving to Las Cruces or some other place to get to a birth, I would end up speeding. I would have my oxygen tanks, and my bags that held everything I could possibly need for a delivery stowed in the back seat of the car. The county sheriff and state police were the ones out in the rural areas who stopped me.

"I am going to a birth," I would say. "Come on with me and help. I don't have anyone with me." They would answer, "Oh, no, lady, we will give you an escort, but we are not going in, that's for sure."

One time I was in my birthing center in Anthony doing prenatal care. A policeman came running in yelling, "Where is she? Where is she?" I could hear him from the back room, where I had a patient on the table listening to heart tones. The waiting room was full of people. I went to the door. He said, "Come with me! Come with me. Get your bag. Come with me."

I tried to question him, but he insisted I go with him right now. I just left the whole place wide open with all the people sitting there. He put me in the squad car and we drove to the Greyhound bus station. He had received a call that a lady at the Greyhound station was having a baby.

She was having contractions five minutes apart and we had plenty of time to transport her to the hospital, but he was not going to see about her without having the midwife with him. They could run into burning buildings and deal with having gunfights in the alley, but no babies.

As time passed I knew all the officers. They got to the point where they did not stop me for love nor money. They would just wave. They did not want any part of what I was up to.

I loved camping. When I felt I could get away, I would go up to Caballo Lake. I would tell my patients who were close to delivery, if they got three contractions in a row, even if they were half an hour apart, to call me. That way I would know if I needed to return immediately.

I would be up at the lake and by the time I would get back into town for a patient, three different people knew that I was speeding on the highway. They all knew my little red station wagon and they always knew who was next in line for delivery.

I just loved the women. They were wonderful. The less money they had, the more hard working and the more responsible they were.

I was not making much money, but I felt that I could not work another regular job or work some place part-time. I wanted to be available to these women. I was a midwife and I felt it strongly in my bones. I knew a lot of midwives who were not willing to ask for money. They did not have it clear in their minds that their services were valuable and that they had a right to ask for money.

I asked for money. A lot of times, I did not get it. I would tell them that they would have to work out some kind of an arrangement with me for minimum wage. They could have their husbands do yard work, they could come over and wash my windows, they could clean the birthing center or do the laundry from the births. They would come in when I had a birth and do cleanups with me or cook for me. Anything to make an equitable exchange where they felt like they were really contributing to the cost of having their baby. We kept track of it by how many hours they spent doing different things.

I had the cleanest windows and the cleanest office. It was way overdone. I was trading out services to meet their needs more than mine. Most of the women were incredibly responsible. The ones who were working in the fields, would literally walk three or four miles, not just for their prenatal visits, but on Fridays to give me that five dollars towards their baby before they spent it.

I was charging $150 per delivery, including all their prenatal care, the delivery, and three months of baby care afterward. That was the indigent sliding scale. If they had money, I was charging $300 total. It was a very good deal. I think probably the going rate at that time was $450 to $500 for prenatal care and delivery by an obstetrician. The hospital bill was extra.

I had foolishly signed only a one-year lease on my birthing center building. After I had done all that work on it and the year was up, the owner let her daughter move into it. By this time, I was licensed in the State of New Mexico. I found a great place in La Mesa, New Mexico. It was two old adobe houses that had been joined together to form one big house. One side I used as office and birthing center. The other side is where my son, Jay, and I lived.

Also, I was doing free prenatal care in Anthony. I paid $20 every Wednesday to rent one room at a real estate office in order to offer free prenatal care. It was an extra big room. I was able to do the prenatal care plus it was large enough to teach Lamaze Childbirth Preparation Classes in Spanish. One of the women who was delivering with me was a native with Spanish as her first language. She helped me teach the class. I was pretty fluent in Spanish in terms of nutrition and questions that had to do with prenatal and deliveries. I needed some assistance in making sure I was using the correct words for exercises and breathing techniques.

The mayor of Sunland Park, New Mexico, offered me a little building for use as a free weekly prenatal site. On Mondays, I would drag along one of my midwife students or one of the doctors from La Clinica who was rotating through my clinics. We did no advertising, but we would have a line of people. It was just a one-room place and they had to stand in the sun or wait in their cars until I called them in.

In order to receive free prenatal care, the women had to sign a contract. It was a simple paper that said they understood I could not accept them as clients or deliver their babies unless they were able to obtain the state required labs and doctor visits. Some of them could not read their own language. I would have to read it to them in Spanish. Few of these women were able to get together enough money to get their lab tests and doctor visits done before their due date.

Only when this was completed could they sign a contract to officially become my client. The vast majority of these women were not going to deliver with me because they did not have the money. The labs and doctor visits were required by New Mexico state law in order for me to deliver them. So they just kept coming for the free prenatal care.

I would do the prenatal care and give them carbon copies of all their records. When they went to the hospital for delivery, they would be able to show they had had prenatal care. The nurses in labor and delivery at Memorial Medical Center in Las Cruces were happy to have these records containing baseline information. Someone showing up in labor with a blood pressure of 120/80 looks perfectly normal unless their records show their average blood pressure through pregnancy had been 100/60. These 'walk-ins' with records made the nurse's job easier and it was much safer for the patient. They were just so grateful to know that their babies were doing fine.

I bought rice and beans in great big sacks, to distribute because their nutrition was so poor. I found out that that did not work. They would take the rice and beans and feed their other children.

The food Co-op in Las Cruces sold an awful tasting protein powder. The kids would not drink it, so the mothers would. I asked my anglo women patients who had money if they would contribute to these women who did not have anything. They would go to the Co-op, buy a box and bring it to me.

I was an early WIC program. I hooked up the women who could get transportation to El Paso or Las Cruces with the actual WIC (Women Infants and Children) federal food program, which was in its infancy and not doing much in the rural areas yet.

I also offered three months of free postpartum and newborn assessments for those women who had not delivered with me, just like I did with my regular clients. It was wonderful to see all the healthy babies and hear the stories of their hospital births.

Whenever I had a concern about the pregnancy of one of my regular client's, I referred her back the doctor who had seen her for her initial assessment. I usually managed to attend the appointments with her so we could all talk together. I developed a good working relationship with the doctors in Anthony and the one in El Paso. By this time a couple of helpful younger OB/GYN's, Marco Duarte and Gene Love, were practicing in Las Cruces.

Upon finding any kind of real health problem in my indigent non-client women, I wrote down all of my findings and instructed them to go to the emergency room at the hospital and present their record copies. It was a county hospital and the ER was required to see anyone who showed up with problems. After an emergency room visit, they were often assigned to a staff obstetrician for crisis intervention care for the rest of their pregnancy.

I felt I had excellent community support. The local newspaper ran a story about my center and practice.

The El Paso Times   Sunday January 3, 1982   Southwest

Old Ways Find New Life In Growing Midwife Trend

By JOAN MORRIS Times staff writer
LAS CRUCES—Kristopher, who will be 3 years old in three months, chewed determinedly on the arm of a plastic galactic storm trooper and gazed wondrously at his new baby brother, looking forward to playing Star Wars with him.

This wasn't their first meeting. Kristopher had been introduced to Michael less than 30 minutes after the infant was born. Michael came rather quickly into the world at the hands of a registered midwife in the bedroom of his parents home.

Kelly and Leslie Greiner of Las Cruces are among a growing number of couples who are opting for home births, shunning the sterile coldness of hospital delivery rooms.

Michael was born Dec. 17, and on his birth certificate, the name of Judy Lee appears as the person responsible for Michael's safe arrival. Ms. Lee is a state-registered midwife whose business has been growing by leaps and bounds during the last year.

Ms. Lee operates Birthways in Las Cruces and in the rural areas of Dona Ana County. The center offers natural childbirth classes and home deliveries for women whose health is good enough to make having a baby at home safe.

State laws regulate midwifery throughout New Mexico, requiring midwives to complete training to receive a state license. Recently, the New Mexico laws were lauded as some of the safest and most progressive regulations in the country.

The move toward home births comes on the heels of a return-to-basics attitude that swept the nation in the late 1960's. Having babies without anesthetic and with the mother being full awake during the birth gave way to so-called natural births where father and family joined in the delivery.

Lately, more and more women are turning to homebirths as a way to save money and to experience what Ms. Lee called the ultimate birth experience. The baby is born at home, into a web of security that some people believe affects the emotional and mental future of the child.

The Greiners recently moved to Las Cruces from North Dakota. Kristopher had been born at the Southwest Maternity Center in Albuquerque, which offers midwife-assisted births in a hospital-like setting. Ms. Greiner said she considered driving to Albuquerque from North Dakota to have Michael. But the Greiners, who have family in Las Cruces, came here instead.

"We just didn't want to have our baby in a hospital," Greiner said. "It just seems too impersonal. We didn't feel comfortable with it." Ms. Greiner said she knew she was healthy and felt like she would be more relaxed having her baby in her own home.

And so, when Ms. Greiner started labor one evening two weeks ago, she called Ms. Lee. When the phone call came that Ms. Greiner was in labor, Ms. Lee was in the shower. She joked later that the birth was so fast that if she had stopped to dry her hair, the Greiners may have had to deliver Michael by themselves.

"I was only in labor about an hour and 37 minutes," Ms. Greiner said, her eyes widening at the speed of Michael's birth. "Judy got here, checked me, and then eight minutes later, there was our new son."

The Greiners had intended to have Kristopher present

to witness the birth of his new brother—although at the time, everyone was convinced it was going to be Kristopher's new sister. But the youngster proved too much for the soon-to-be new parents.

"He was really excited and he kept jumping up and down on the bed," Ms. Greiner said. "Finally, I just had to send him to his grandmother's." Ms. Greiner said she wanted Kristopher to feel like he, too, was part of the birth. "I didn't want to send him to his grandmother's and then have him come back the next morning with a new brother in the family," she said.

So after Michael was born, Kristopher and all the in-laws came over to see the new baby. Ms. Greiner said her mother-in-law had six children, but had never really seen a birth or the processes that come after. She said the woman thanked her for allowing her to share in Michael's beginning.

Michael arrived shortly after 9 p.m. Dec. 17. He weighed just 1 ounce shy of 7 pounds. Greiner bragged that Michael didn't cry, but just kind of looked around as if to get acquainted with his new home. Greiner also said both Kristopher and Michael were exceptional babies who sleep through the night and don't cry all the time.

The Greiners said they would recommend home births for everyone, but warned that not everyone is healthy enough nor would they feel comfortable with having a baby at home. Ms. Greiner said women should ask around and find out if home delivery is for them. She said some women feel more secure in a hospital and probably would have a difficult time having a baby at home.

"But I just wouldn't like having my baby in a hospital," she said. "When you have a baby at home, you realize right from the start that the responsibility for taking care of the kid is yours, and not some nurse's who does this all the time. You get to wash him, feed him and clothe him for the first time. It all sinks in and it isn't frightening anymore."

The Greiners said while having a baby with a midwife in attendance is a lot cheaper than with a doctor in a hospital, the cost had nothing to do with their decision. "You aren't sick when you are having a baby, so I don't see why you should be in a hospital," Ms. Greiner said. "Even if having a baby at home cost twice as much as having one in a hospital, we still would do it this way."

The Greiners said they don't plan to have any more children. "I missed my chance for a girl," Ms. Greiner said. "Now it's going to be just me and the Greiner guys."

Joan Morris, a journalist for the *El Paso Times*, came to me to talk about writing a story about home birth. The Greiners are the ones she decided to do the story about. She was very supportive and wrote stories that were objective and unbiased.

She did not want to develop any kind of personal relationship with me because she felt it would destroy her objectivity and credibility in writing other stories. Earlier Joan had attemped to use the newspaper to educate the public about midwives, our education and state rules for practice.

The El Paso Times Sun Aug 16, 1981 New Mexico Edition

NM Law Requires Midwives To Keep Trained And Be Reviewed

LAS CRUCES—There are 23 pages of regulations, qualifications, and dos and don'ts in New Mexico's laws governing midwifery. The regulations set up criteria for who may become a midwife as well as establish review procedures and registration revocation.

According to the regulations, only persons registered as lay midwives can assist regularly with home deliveries. To become a midwife, persons must have completed as least four years of high school or the equivalent, a course in the theory of pregnancy and childbirth, clinical training (usually a six months course), a state Health Services Division course in prenatal nutrition, a course in prepared childbirth for the home birth setting, and a course in cardiopulmonary resuscitation of the mother and newborn.

They must have a doctor's statement certifying the absence of any communicable disease, must have four recommendations, and must pay a $50 fee.

Registration as a midwife is completed after the person passes a written and oral exam administered by a midwifery board. Registration also must be renewed each year. Practicing lay midwives must obtain eight hours of continuing education before the registration is renewed.

The midwife must require the patient to have a risk evaluation and physical examination by a physician before a registered lay midwife assumes her care, the regulations state. According to the regulations, a woman must have one prenatal visit with a physician when she is between 36 and 40 weeks pregnant.

After the baby is born, the mother must take the child to a doctor for examination within three days.

Midwives are forbidden to take as patients women with uncontrolled high blood pressure; women who develop swelling in the face and hands; have severe and persistent headaches or visual disturbances; women who do not gain 14 pounds by the end of the 30th gestation week; and women who have symptoms of vaginitis, urinary tract infection, vaginal bleeding before labor, or premature rupture of membranes.

During the delivery, if the midwife detects any irregularities, she is required by law to refer the woman to a doctor for immediate attention. There are an additional 22 restrictions on the type of women who may have a home delivery. –JOAN MORRIS

La Clinica de Familia

La Clinica de Familia is a rural federal health initiative program in the southern part of New Mexico. Back then, their doctors were Family Practice physicians. Most of my Hispanic women were already patients of La Clinica.

In the Hispanic population, home birth and midwives are the traditional way of having babies. They really did not want to go to the hospital. They would come to me for care but they had to have the doctor involved at some juncture within the pregnancy.

The doctor would check them, review the chart and certify they were not high risk. They had to have another visit after 36 weeks of pregnancy.

Mary Banes, the Executive Director, ran a really tight ship. She made sure I was properly introduced to their new Medical Director, Dr. David Nolting. I developed a good working relationship with him since we were both doing four or five births a month.

Dr. Nolting performed a lot of the required exams and was impressed with my meticulous record keeping. I had my instructor, Shari Daniels, to thank for that. She was tougher than a marine drill sergeant.

I did not hesitate to refer patients back to him if I had a concern or a problem. He could order ultrasounds, a service that was offered through the rural health initiative program with federal monies. It did not cost the patient a fortune.

Rotating through their clinics were physicians in residency training for Family Practice Specialty. Dr. Nolting liked what I was doing and heard good things from the patients. He started sending his residents to spend five or six days at the birthing center observing what we did.

He was the one who suggested it. He told me about the

Family Practice residents rotating through La Clinica, and he wanted them to rotate through my center. He would also have three or four residents at one time, from places like University New Mexico, Stanford, and Harvard. Each resident would rotate through my clinic a week at a time.

It was such fun to see these doctors come into my carpeted birthing center. How could I possibly do deliveries here? Of course, the birthing room had tile floors and could be easily cleaned and sanitized.

I usually had a student midwife doing rotations along with the residents. She was the lead person. I was the other lead person. I would review the records and say, "Okay, she had low growth or slow growth and we need to make sure that the fundus is accurately measured. If there is any question about it, you need to call me in on her visit." The big question for the doctor performing the prenatal visit was, does the woman speak any English?

I went back and forth between English and Spanish all day long on the phone and in person. I could never remember if they spoke Spanish or English. I would say, "It is written on the chart. On the intake on the chart it says, "SSO, Spanish speaking only." I would be talking Spanish on the phone and English to the residents and somebody else in the room would ask me something in Spanish. Suddenly, I realized that I had become quite bilingual.

The doctor rotating through my clinic during the week for prenatal care was on call in the evenings for La Clinica. I would call them to attend the births. They observed and would do dilation checks with me. I would do the dilation checks, have them check behind me and we would compare cervix dilation centimeters.

The residents were all men except for one. The patients were not all that thrilled about having a male doctor do exams on them. The interns were upset when a woman would not let them in the room for a birth or a woman would not allow them to perform an exam. The patient was the decision-maker. I never said, "Hey, this guy is working with me so he gets to touch you." The women who did not want to be examined, usually would allow them to listen to heart tones and do fundal height measurements.

I had a working arrangement with a Family Practice physician in Las Cruces. He found out that I delivered babies over an intact perineum and did not have perineal tears. He did not know how to deliver a baby without cutting an episiotomy. He called and asked if I would arrange for him to attend a couple of births so that he could see a delivery over an intact perineum. Also, he wanted to be certain that none of his peers knew he was coming to learn from me. It was all hush-hush.

I had a hell of a time persuading any of the women to allow him to attend. His nose was out of joint. "Well, just tell them that I am going to come. I am not going to charge them."

I explained, "They don't care if you are not going to charge them. They want a woman provider. They don't want a man."

It turned out that the one woman who allowed him to be a guest was all set up to deliver in her bed in the bedroom. At the last minute, she decided she wanted to deliver on the living room floor. We put a sheet under her and a couple of Chux pads and allowed her to deliver on the living room floor. We had the oxygen tanks and the IV's ready to go if needed. The doc was shocked and upset over this sudden change of plans.

We applied hot compresses and massaged with olive oil, and patiently waited for the contractions to expand the perineum. It was peaceful and gentle, no rush for the next push. The birth proceeded: the slow delivery of the head; the rotation of the baby; wiping the face and gentle suctioning. We kept the water that gushed from the vagina from entering the baby's nose.

After it was over, he was absolutely elated. He had never seen anything like this in his training. He was very impressed.

Two of the resident physicians doing the rotations through my clinic went on to have home births themselves. Heaven only knows the impact of the other rotations through my clinic.

I served a great need in the community with support from some of the local physicians and was busy enjoying my practice. I was unaware of the storm hovering, and took little note of

Linda Lonsdale's reference to the "three ring circus" in this December 1981 newspaper article.

The El Paso Times   Wed Dec 9, 1981   Southwest

Midwives In State Gaining Acceptance

By Don Frederick Times staff writer
SANTA FE—New Mexico won praise Tuesday as a nationwide leader in regulations allowing midwives to deliver babies at home.

The publisher of "Mothering" magazine published in Albuquerque, said a state-by-state survey she recently conducted shows New Mexico has the country's "most progressive and innovative" regulating procedure for midwives.

Peggy O'Mara McMahon said that as a result, there is a "national focus" on New Mexico as interest in midwifery grows in other states. Her praise of New Mexico's regulatory process was echoed by midwives attending a meeting conducted by state Health and Environment Department officials. But several midwives also agreed their services have gained greater acceptance in northern than in southern New Mexico.

Tish Dimmin, a member of the state advisory board on midwife regulations, said cooperation by local doctors with midwives ranges from excellent in Taos to good in Santa Fe and Albuquerque to only fair in southern New Mexico.

One of the state's key regulations requires a woman wanting to deliver her baby at home with a registered midwife to have a thorough physical examination by a qualified doctor. The woman must be certified by the doctor as being unlikely to experience medical or psychological problems while giving birth.

Jody Christie, a midwife living in Alamogordo, said only one doctor in the city has been "willing to stick his neck out" and consistently provide examinations for women who have hired her.

Linda Lonsdale, head of the HED office responsible

for regulating midwives, said most of the 40 midwives registered by the state are in the Taos, Santa Fe and Albuquerque areas. Ms. Lonsdale said a few of those registered live in Silver City, Las Cruces and Alamogordo but none are from communities in southeastern New Mexico.

Ms. Lonsdale also said the biggest dispute between local doctors and a midwife that she knows of in the state has occurred in Las Cruces. "That's the only three-ring circus I've run into," she said of the Las Cruces conflict.

The El Paso Times reported in August that the only registered midwife in Las Cruces, Judy Lee, was having difficulty finding local doctors willing to perform the required prenatal examinations of her clients.

At the time, Dr. Braden said he and most other doctors in Las Cruces were refusing to work with Ms. Lee because they oppose midwifery as it is allowed to be practiced in New Mexico.

Braden, contacted Tuesday at his Las Cruces office, said most of the city's medical community still is unwilling to provide examinations for Ms. Lee's clients.

Braden said he thinks midwives can "do an excellent job" working with doctors within a hospital setting. But Braden said he remains opposed to the New Mexico system allowing midwives to deliver babies at home without a doctor present.

Braden also criticized as "inadequate" the educational requirements a person must fulfill before being registered as a midwife.

Ms. Lee said Tuesday that although most Las Cruces doctors still refuse to work with her, "there are a few that I can turn to." She added her business is "excellent".

So we helped to change the home birth climate in other states. Even today, this gives me a great sense of satisfaction.

During this time I was a member of a study group at New Mexico State University. It was comprised of 15 people including members from La Clinica's administration. I was recruited because I had delivered the baby of one of the women who was on the committee. We were putting together a proposal to apply to the federal government for a grant for teen pregnancy prevention. The university provided us with a professional grant writer. I was a community resource for identifying problems and barriers to the delivery of prenatal care to the indigent. I was the only one doing free prenatal care in the county.

We met regularly for four months in order to finish the grant application. It made sense that the monies would be distributed by La Clinica, because they already had the facilities and personnel to provide the services.

That year the federal government funded only three sites in the whole nation. We were one of them. We received this grant of hundreds of thousands of dollars based on our terrible statistics for infant mortality, lack of prenatal care, and high teen pregnancy rates.

When the monies were finally ready to come down, all kinds of paper work was required. The doctors at La Clinica were Family Practice physicians. The federal government required that they have a written contract with the obstetricians in Las Cruces agreeing that they would do their cesarean section deliveries and emergency services.

Dr. Murray Bruder told La Clinica if they supported the midwife or had any kind of working relationship with me, he would not let any of the doctors in town sign off on this grant. La Clinica and the community stood to lose thousands of dollars from the grant. He forced La Clinica to stop their cooperative effort with me.

I understood how awful the doctors and the Board at La Clinica felt. They did not want to tell me that they could not have a professional relationship with me anymore. They were between a rock and a hard place.

I totally understood that they would not see any of my patients anymore, that I could not refer any patients to them. Then I started to think about this and realized what Bruder and his partner, Braden, were doing to La Clinica was extortion.

Here were huge amounts of money the community desperately needed for teen pregnancy and they were going to hold that money hostage. And yes, they dumped me. What else could they do?

I did have support within the community, but I was not prepared for what followed.

START WITH 10,000 BONUS MILES

A Gold Delta SkyMiles® Credit Card can make your SkyMiles® balance take-off!

Apply today:

americanexpress.com/goldoffers

1-800-395-8000

BOARDING PASS

******* ET *******

ANDERSON/THOMASWARRE

SEAT
108

20:8 ?

FLIGHT	DATE
OLSZ25	20SEP

ORIGIN
ST GEORGE UTAH

DESTINATION
SALT LAKE CITY

OPERATED BY SKYWEST AIRLINES
A DELTA CONNECTION CARRIER

The Struggle Begins

I guess what started first was the doctors refusing to give my women copies of their records and refusing to send copies to me. Among my patients were several women professors and professors' wives from the university. Their private insurance companies had started reimbursing me.

These were intelligent women that had the guts to say something. They started demanding their records. When they were refused, they demanded the reason be put in writing. The physicians writing letters on their own letterhead, said it was dangerous to go to a midwife. They further threatened them by saying they could not return to the physician for birth control pills or pap tests or any other type of health care.

It was my feeling at the time, and still today, that nobody was pissed off until I started processing insurance claims, and making some money. The doctors' attitude was it was okay if I only took care of migrant workers who could not afford to pay me anyhow—not really okay—but not financially worrisome.

Then I had a postpartum transport to Memorial Medical Center, the hospital in Las Cruces. After the delivery, I had examined the placenta. A piece of the placenta about the size of a nickel was missing. Her bleeding was normal, but I was so cautious that I decided that I had better take her into the hospital and get one of the doctors to take a look. They made us wait and wait and wait in this room. They would not let the lady go pee. We are talking about the danger of postpartum hemorrhage here, and the risk of postpartum hemorrhage is increased by a full bladder.

I knew the nurse assigned to us. I just knew she was trying to tell us something. She would come into the room and make funny motions. I did not understand at first, but suddenly I snapped to it. She was trying to tell me nonverbally that the conversations between me and the husband and the wife were being monitored on the intercom at the nurse's station. After she was out of the room, I said "What the hell, let's just pull out one of these drawers and pee in it. Fuck 'em." I pulled out the drawer on the exam table, and man, the nurses were in there immediately to take her to the bathroom.

Later, this patient wrote a letter to the Board of Directors of the hospital complaining about the treatment she received.

October 7, 1981

. . . upon arrival at the hospital I was not examined by a doctor for over 2 hours although a doctor was present in the ER throughout this period of time. Despite having never seen me Dr. Phillips, the obstetrician, ordered an IV with Pitocin [a drug to reduce uterine bleeding]. Repeated requests for permission to use the restroom or a bedpan were ignored. . . I was then informed, without being examined, that it was necessary to remove the placenta pieces by surgery. I was subsequently kept overnight and through the next day in complete disregard of the needs of my newborn infant, from whom I was separated during this time. . . Judy Lee was denied access to the operating room when I specifically requested her presence. New Mexico HED-80-3 Regulations governing the Practice of Lay Midwifery state, in Section 811, "The midwife must accompany the mother and should remain to ascertain outcome." A personal letter from Richard Perkins, M.D. Perinatologist and OB/GYN Director of the University of New Mexico, regarding Ms. Lee's qualifications to act in this capacity of support/liason, was ignored.

The negative attitude of the doctors towards clients of midwives were later made more apparent to me by an ER staff member's account of a doctor commenting on not wishing to "handle the midwife's leftovers."

Two and a half months later she received a response to her complaint from Kevin Andrews, Hospital Administrator.

December 23, 1981

. . . your concerns were forwarded to the Department of Obstetrics & Gynecology for a thorough medical review by the department members. Their detailed review/analysis of your complaint follows.

In regard to the care rendered to you in the ER the Department of OB/GYN determined: "In the presence of a reliable history of a retained fragment of placenta, the only appropriate course of therapy is examination under general anesthesia and dilatation and curettage of the uterine cavity . . . The analysis went on to indicate that when you arrived in the ER with your midwife, Ms. Lee, in attendance, your problem was immediately identified by the fact that Ms. Lee described the missing fragment of placenta tissue and even brought with her the placenta. In the presence of such a reliable history, the ER appropriately contacted the obstetrician [who was] on call. . . You were not seen by the ER physician because the appropriate consultation had been called and you were not in an acute emergency situation at the moment.

An IV was started, laboratory work initiated, and the Operating Room notified of the necessity for a D & C. If examination had been undertaken in the ER by one of the ER physicians, this would have resulted in excessive manipulation of the uterus, increasing the risk of infection or bleeding. . . Therefore, the Department of OB/GYN concludes that the points made in your letter were excellent questions but medically the treatment ordered and carried out was medically appropriate.

You expressed some concern regarding Ms. Lee's denial of access to the Operating Room when you had specifically requested her presence. . . This denial of access, in the opinion of this institution, has no way compromised Ms. Lee's ability to ascertain the outcome of your care.

[your last]. . . point speaks to the negative attitude of physicians toward clients of midwives. Perceptions are a difficult thing to deal with. However, it's unfortunate that the ER staff member you attribute this comment to has such an influence on your perceptions. The Department of OB/GYN has indicated to me that based upon the excellent treatment they believe you received while a patient in the OB/GYN service, could in no way have demonstrated that there was a negative attitude among care toward clients of midwives. I think it is appropriate to indicate

that if a staff member in the ER was sharing a personal opinion, that was inappropriate. I suggest that you judge the attitude of physicians who care for you based upon the quality of the care given you and not on what someone tells you.
cc: Members of the Board of Directors
Chairman, Department of OB/GYN

This answer appeared to me to be skewed. I am the midwife who is not qualified to enter the Operating Room, yet the treatment plan was made and carried out based on a "most reliable history from Ms. Lee, the midwife".

I started getting protests from insurance companies that had paid me in the past. After that started, I would send in the claim forms with a copy of my license and a copy of the overview of State of New Mexico laws. I included my license number and said, "Pay me."

They added delaying tactics to their claims process. I would talk to the actual claims adjusters, asking what was missing. Their response was, we are getting a lot of flack from your local medical society not to pay you. We have to review these thoroughly. My claims were getting delayed three, four, and six months before being paid.

The group of women from the University got together and wrote letters of protest, putting some powerful pressure on the insurance company. Their message was, "We pay for these benefits and you pay this midwife and don't give us any flack." I think that is when the doctors realized that they were not going to be able to bulldoze me. I had not only my own strong convictions, but I also had educated women with money who were not going to let them ignore me.

Then the obscene phone calls began. Lots of hang up phone calls, which I had never had before. Occasionally the phone would ring and I would answer in English. Then the caller would hang up, call back and try to speak to me in Spanish. Just all kinds of obscene stuff—telling me what they were going to do to me, where they wanted to bite me, lick me, touch me, how hot I was, baby, baby. It was really gross and disgusting stuff.

Sometimes they would ask for Judy Lee like a regular

phone call and then suck me in. There were several people doing it, at least two or three different voices.

I called the sheriff's office about it. They said, "Don't worry about it. These people don't know who you really are. They are getting your name out of a phone book. They are just weirdos. It is probably the same guy and he just got a response from you the first time and he is going for it again."

I knew it was not just one person. It was at home, on my beeper number and on my work number. I did not have secretaries and answering services. I was not making enough money to afford anything better than an answering machine and a beeper. I had to answer the phone. It happened at all hours of the day, middle of the afternoon, at three and four in the morning. I just never knew. It was one thing to have your sleep interrupted for patients, but this really kept me from getting any rest, as well as constantly upsetting me.

I attempted again to get help from the deputy sheriff's office. I told them that I did not think their explanation was correct. I asked them what could be done. Back then I guess it was a really big deal to try to trace phone calls. Either that or they just were not that interested.

Then I noticed a little change in the level of the volume on the phone line. The first time I heard it I knew what it was. But I thought, no, I am paranoid. I am just crazy because of all the obscene calls. I waited maybe four days, but I knew it was a tap on the phone. Back in Chicago my dad worked for the phone company. He put taps on our home phones on a periodic basis to see what we teenagers were up to. You would hear this slight little change in volume, no clicks or anything.

I finally persuaded the sheriff's deputy to come and check my phone. He thought I was crazy, but indulged me. I guess he thought by checking the house and all the phone wires he would get me off his back. He found no problem. Three days later, I called them back, insisting something was definitely there. They again explained they had checked all the wires at the house and nothing was wrong with my phone.

I remembered my father used to tap phones directly at the phone company. I asked if the deputy would have it checked by the men from the telephone company. The deputy asked me why I would have a criminal wire tap on my phone? I answered that I had no idea but that something was definitely going on.

I do not know what made him believe me, but the telephone company sent out a service man to check. He actually climbed the phone poles. He traced the lines back several telephone poles from my house. Three poles down the road from my house he found a tap.

The deputy returned and apologized. "You are absolutely right. The phone company just found this tap and it is a professional job. This is not someone kidding around." I thanked him and his partner. I asked what they were going to do about it. The phone company had removed the tap and said it was a criminal matter. People could not be trespassing on the phone company's poles. I think the deputy sheriff and the phone company were shocked that I was right.

I was glad the tap was off the phone. Afterwards, I never even thought about who would have done it or why. I do not know why I did not take it more seriously. I just went about my business. The obscene phone calls stopped. Getting the police involved was a good idea.

Everything was normal for several weeks. Then I heard the tap back on the phone. And the obscene phone calls began again. I called the sheriff's office. The deputy came out with the phone crew and found and removed another tap device from the same pole where it was located before. At the time, I was busy delivering babies, taking care of my moms and dealing with all the political stuff. I was not taking care of myself and was denying my fears.

I kept getting the obscene phone calls at all hours of the day and night. I never had more than an hour or so of unbroken sleep. Then the obscene phone calls were from just one voice, a guy. He was talking very personally. I realized that he knew who I was. He knew where I worked and was telling me stuff about myself.

One day the caller told me, "Yeah, you were really looking hot at Albertson's in that red dress." I had on a red dress and had bought groceries at Albertson's that day. I was really getting panicky. I was afraid to open the door if a man came to the door of my office and I did not recognize him as a husband of a patient.

Two weeks later, the same little obscure noise returned to my phone. The same policeman and the same phone lineman came to check. The officer came back to talk to me. He was a detective. He said that they had found a device again, further away and well hidden. Again, it was thought to be done by a professional.

(With the recall of these events during the interview, Judy was shaking so badly, we had to take a few minutes for her to do some deep breathing and relaxation techniques before we could go on.)

I explained that I just did not understand. He practically throttled me. He was irritated that I was so naive that I did not get it. I just remember the smell of the honeysuckle in the air and standing on that porch in the dark and him urging me to think. He could not know who had the motive to do this, but he felt that I did. He explained it was a professional job that did not come cheap. He questioned me about who would be motivated to put me out of business.

I was in shock at the time. I could hardly stand when it dawned on me how serious these people were. That is when I knew the obscene phone call person was part of this, trying to scare me so badly that I would be unfocused with my women. Losing sleep from receiving anonymous phone calls all hours during the night, I would do something stupid from lack of sleep.

I was afraid to go out, either in day time or at night. I never, ever prior to this was politically active. I was a feminist but a quiet one. I went to meetings and supported where needed, but I never marched in demonstrations. I always avoided this kind of activity. Then all of a sudden, I was having to defend myself and defend my women. I started the search to hire an attorney to make my defense official.

Stephen A. Hubert was the only lawyer in Las Cruces who had ever sued the hospital. Nobody else in the community would take any clients for legal action against the hospital. I went to see him.

I explained the crazy situation: the letters that these doctors were giving their women saying that they could not have any more babies with them; threatening my women that if anything happened, they would not go to the hospital to take care of them; telling them it was dangerous to have a midwife home birth; refusing to allow them to return to get birth control pills after having a midwife delivery. I explained what happened with LaClinica and my back-up getting pulled, the obscene phone calls, and the illegal wire taps discovered on the phone.

The lawyer called this restraint of trade, collusion and harassment. He knew all the right words to assign to it. I only knew what I was experiencing.

His response surprised me. "I have absolutely no experience with this. You are right, you need somebody that will go to bat for you. And I am assuming that you don't have any money."

"Right," I answered. "I am actually getting insurance payments for some of my women, but the majority pay me in chickens or yard work."

It did not faze him. He was really a good guy. He said he would call around the United States and find out who knew about anti-trust and restraint of trade. It was a super-specialized area.

A couple of weeks later, he had contacted a law firm out of Tuscon, Arizona. One of their lawyers called me long distance. Their message was, "We have done this kind of thing before. We know you don't have any money. If there is any money to be made out of this, we are going to take half of it. I think that what we can do is scare the shit out of these guys and they will back off if this is okay with you." I responded that I had no interest in law suits, but I needed the harrassment to stop.

Up until this point, I had two wondereful obstetricians in Las Cruces who were doing back up for me, Dr. Gene Love and Dr. Marco Duarte. My agreement with them was if they ever had to do a cesarean section on one of my patients, I would pay their fee myself. I could not pay the hospital bill. It was a county and city hospital and my indigent women had some recourse to health care funds if they were unable to pay the hospital charges.

I called on Drs. Love and Durarte only for problems with patients that I planned to deliver. They were not committed to doing anything with any of the women who were receiving free prenatal care from me. These women would show up at the emergency room as walk-ins.

I served on several state committees that dealt with medical services within the community. One was a brand new committee which looked at medical "certificates of need". I heard they were soliciting health care providers within the county to be on the board, as well as private citizens. I filled out a written application and sent a resume. They accepted me.

It was set up so that we all started out on equal footing with an equal say. One member of the board was a paid staff person. Whenever a medical institution or a practice wanted to begin a new medical process or increase the number of hospital beds in an area, the staff person would do an analysis of the project, and then we would have meetings to discuss its need. The needs we dealt with were advertised x-ray machines, MRI equipment, and who could perform physical rehabilitation services—services that were related to health issues.

The board was comprised of citizens and doctors mostly. I was the only midwife. Bruder was also on this board. My membership was something that kind of stuck in Dr. Bruder's craw. He was the head of the county medical association and I had equal vote and say on the committee with him. He would always make it a point to sit as far away from me as possible. If at all possible, he would have somebody else ask me a question rather than addressing me himself. I am sure that if Bruder had had any say in the membership of this group, I would not have been appointed.

The meetings were held in Truth or Consequences, New Mexico, an hour's drive north. With all the obscene phone calls and threats coming in, I really was concerned about attending the meetings. They were in the evenings and lasted until nine or ten o'clock.

I started taking a friend with me. We would drive up in the after the the afternoon, have early dinner, and I would attend the evening meeting. My friend would just sit out in the parking

One of my free prenatal care patients missed three con-

lot and take a nap and then be with me on the drive back home.

One of my free prenatal care patients missed three consecutive appointments at the end of her pregnancy. I assumed she had delivered. Then she appeared at my clinic undelivered. I asked her where she had been. She replied she had just been waiting each day to have the baby. She had no complaints, but her blood pressure was dangerously high. Not only were her hands and feet swollen, but so were her legs and face. She was obviously pre-eclamptic and past her due date—a serious condition.

Her baby's heart tones sounded strong and regular. I warned her that she and the baby could be in terrible trouble if she did not get professional attention immediately. Even though she said that she "looked like this with her other pregnancies", I told her again how dangerous it could be for her and the baby. I was trying to convince her to go to the hospital immediately, not to wait until she went into labor. She replied that she was not in the country legally and was afraid she would be deported. I told her that she could end up dead or with a dead baby. I tried to explain that deportation was not as bad as a dead baby. I felt terrible talking to her like that but I knew she needed immediate medical attention and there was nothing I personally could do for her.

I wrote my findings and my advice to her on her records and reminded her to take the carbon copy of her previous visits. She did go to the hospital right away. She received appropriate high risk care and, thankfully, she and the baby were fine.

The next day I got a phone call from Santa Fe. They said that there had been a complaint against me by Dr. Murray Bruder, the head doctor at the hospital. Apparenty, I had let one of my patients become dangerously toxemic and had handled the situation improperly. I tried to explain what had happened, but she would not listen.

She informed me that my license was suspended immediately. The woman said that I was accused of accepting high risk patients and these women had not had their lab tests done nor been seen by a doctor. Although I was in total shock, I tried to explain that these women were not my patients. I was only providing free prenatal and postpartum care.

Both the patient and I had signed papers in Spanish, that were read aloud to them, if they could not read. The form explicitly said that they understood I could not accept them as patients unless or until they were able to meet certain conditions. The paper also clearly said that I definitely would not deliver their babies and that they had to make other arrangements with the hospital or elsewhere for their births.

I pleaded that I had women who were due to deliver and that I needed time to communicate with them. I needed time to find another midwife to cover for me. All to no avail. My license was suspended immediately. They would explain it to me in writing and some kind of trial would be scheduled later.

Although I was in a state of shock, I immediately got on the phone trying to find another midwife to cover the deliveries that were due. Jodie Christie was the first to say she would help me. She was in Alamogordo, New Mexico, which was an hour and a half drive. This was generous of her because she also had women due. We were both in a panic about what had happened. She and the midwives in El Paso were aware that I had been doing free care for many months.

Shari Daniels, Director of The Maternity Center in El Paso, also agreed to see all my patients and deliver them during this crisis. But she was doing between 30 and 40 births a month at the center, and my patients would have to somehow manage to get down to The Maternity Center in the Segundo Barrio of El Paso. Shari's students who had been working with me, had not yet sat for their licensing exams. They could help but not actually provide services without on-site supervision. We all wondered aloud, "How could the state just call and suspend my license on the spot when all I did was appropriately refer a woman in trouble for the care she needed?"

Once Jodie and Shari agreed they would cover for me as best they could, considering the significant distance, I started calling my women who were due to deliver. I cried as I told them the bad news.

They were upset. They knew and trusted me and my students. They had never met Jodie. I reassured them that I would be at their births as a support person if I was not arrested. That was still up in the air. The state did not tell me what was happening or how it would play out. All my "pregos", as I called them, were very supportive and wanted to do whatever they could to help. I had no idea what could be done, but was grateful for their offering.

One of the patients I called that day was a student at the university. She was absolutely furious. At first I thought she was angry at me. When I explained the situation further she said, "they can't just pull your license without a hearing first." I explained that I had tried to tell them that I had women due. I could have explained everything if they would have only listened. But they would not listen. I told her exactly what they said: "We can, and have, already pulled your license."

I could not deliver any woman nor provide any more care until after the hearing or trial. My student patient was still furious. She asked me for the phone number. She instructed me, "Do not make any more calls. Just stay there and my dad will call you right away." I had never met her father. She was an out-of-state student.

Within five minutes her father called me. He was an attorney. He calmly asked if he might try to help me out in this matter, because it was illegal for the state to suspend my license without a hearing, unless, of course, I killed somebody or something similarly heinous. I told him what had transpired. He asked the name of the person who had called and my permission to call them back on my behalf. Well, I was thrilled that he would try to do something for me.

A short time later I got a call from the state. They said they had decided I could keep practicing until after the hearing. I breathed a sigh of relief. They informed me the hearing would be scheduled in Santa Fe within the next 30 days. My immediate response was, "Why can't the hearing be held in Dona Ana County? This is where I practice and I have lots of babies due." They said it could not be done. I was just so happy to have my license back, I did not argue the point.

I called my student prego who had intervened. We laughed and cried together over what her dad had been able to accomplish with one little phone call, and he was not even licensed in New Mexico! He also advised that I get myself an attorney right away. How was I going to manage that, with no money? But, at least I was still able to practice.

I immediately called Jodie, telling her to spread the word to the other midwives while I called my women to say it had been a false alarm. Then I sat down and prayed and gave thanks. Once again guardian angels had intervened and watched over me and my women.

The thing that confused me was the fact that the director, who provided supervision and oversight for the state regulations of midwifery services, and I had had an excellent relationship up to this point. We had regular conversations about my work with student midwives. She knew all about the free clinics I was holding. I had even showed her most of the disclaimer paperwork I was using to tell the women what they had to do before I could accept them as my own clients. She knew how the labor and delivery nurses had responded so positively. I even sent her photos of the two freebie locations in Anthony and Sunland Park. I was so proud of what we were able to do for these women.

The pharmacist, Mr. Palafox, Mayor Baca, La Clinica de Familia Medical Director, Dr. David Nolting, and many others in all three communities, knew me by name. They all made referrals of women in need. Nothing was secret. If it were something I should not have been doing, why in the world would I give women copies of their records to take with them to the hospital?

As the legal and media battle unfolded, I did continue to work. During this time, I had had a couple of run-ins associated with transports to the hospital of women who were not going to deliver with me. I did not have Non-stress Test equipment, so Iwould have the mother drink orange juice, which would give the baby a kick of sugar, and perform a manual check for number of baby movements during the next twenty minutes. If the baby did not move normal during this time frame, I would send the mother to the hospital with a note stating that this woman is reporting less fetal activity than usual. I included the findings of my manual test and copies of all her other records.

The emergency room doctor would send them to the OB on call.

When I had to send a woman who was going to deliver with me, I would actually travel with her to the hospital. No serious problems, mostly, they had failure to progress, or were dehydrated. They were usually women with insurance. They would ask for the same doctor they had seen for their prenatal reviews. Other women were assigned to whoever was on call.

Several times that turned out to be Dr. Braden, who was Dr. Bruder's older partner. This guy at times would be drunk as a skunk. He would come to the hospital smelling like booze. The accepted rumor about this behavior was, "Oh, he just takes a lot of allergy medicine."

I complained about it to the nurses to no avail. They had tried everything to get him to stop practicing—going as far as taking complaints to Santa Fe. Obviously, doctors were not reprimanded on complaints from nursing staff. More Politics! The little folks were losing, yet again.

One night, I was at the hospital with one of my women who was going to have a C-section. Dr. Braden came in on call and was literally bumping into walls. I said to the nurses that he could absolutely not perform surgery on my patient. I stood in the doorway and would not allow the nurses to place her on the stretcher if he was going to be the one operating. The nurses threatened to get the hospital administrator.

My reponse was, "Get whoever you want here. But this ain't gonna happen. This guy is not going to cut on my woman. We will take a chance on whatever happens, but he is not going to be the one who does this surgery." The nurses called Bruder to cover for Braden. Bruder did the C-section.

Some time after this incident, Braden resigned and retired from obstetrics. There was never any investigation by the hospital. There was no kind of stink or disgrace associated with Braden retiring. It was handled as though he was old and decided to retire from delivering babies. He continued his private practice as a gynecologist.

(Author's Note: During the time I was doing research for a book of birth stories from women in the community, I encountered two

birth stories from mothers who knew Judy Lee. The following is an inter-
view with a former employee of the hospital who had worked in labor and
delivery. At the time of the interview, she did not know that I was writing
Judy Lee's story.)

I worked there as a nurse in Labor and Delivery. I left
the hospital in 1980. Dr. Love, who was my doctor,
was awesome. The main reason I went to him to have
my baby, though, is because I didn't want to go with
one of the other doctors. I knew all the docs from
working with them. For example, if you went to Dr.
Duarte, who was nice, you had a chance of getting
Bruder. At the time, they were practicing together.

Q   You left labor and delivery in 1980?
A   Yes. I went to work for a surgeon.

Q   I am writing another book about a Licensed Midwife
       who started a birth center here in Dona County in
       the late 1970's and Bruder reported her to the Mid-
       wifery Regulation Board and tried to get her license
       revoked. Do you remember that?
A   Yes, I do.

Q   You are the first person that I have come across that
       remembered anything about it? Do you mind talk-
       ing about it?
A   No problem. It really wasn't so much Braden. Be-
       cause Braden drank. He was a nice man. He adopted
twenty kids and put them through college. He was
actually a good man.

Bruder was the one who defamed her. He would put
it out about all these critical, bad deliveries that can
happen at home and why you need an obstetrician. If
any of the women that came to them were even interested in a midwife, he would give them horror stories. I have heard him tell horror stories. Back then

he had a big political business base. He had the way to squash her and did. It was really Bruder.

Q   It wasn't until '82 and '83 that he really went after her?

A   Right, but I still knew the girls in labor and delivery at the hospital. I knew he did some stuff but I didn't know about the phone tapping. I do know that he did a lot of business stuff that just made it impossible for her to survive.

.   She started her practice in 1978 and it was 1985 before she left. So by the time he finished with her, she kind of won. He didn't put her out of business. She just didn't have the energy to carry on.

Dr. Bruder was horrible. He would be in the doctors' surgical lounge bragging. I would be there waiting for surgery with my employer and heard Dr. Bruder talking [about])what he did to try to thwart this midwifery thing. How it was a bunch of quackery. Just bombastic bragging to any nurses and doctors listening.

Q   When we started with the book, Judy was going through some papers and stuff and found all these newspapers that document a lot of what happened. She had obscene phone calls.

A   Yes, I heard about that.

Q   Tell me what you heard?
At the time I did not know that he was talking about the midwife, but later when I heard what happened to her, I put the pieces together and felt it was her. He had people—I can't remember who he said did this—it was not his employees or relatives. But he hired people to call, just random people.

Dr. Love was her backup physician. He was the one she would call when she ran into problems or had a critical case, like a good midwife should. He supported her.

Stephanie Blank was a lawyer involved with La Clinica. She knew that I had been having trouble. She contacted me offering her help with the issue of my license hearing. "I'll do the paperwork for you," she said. "I know you don't have any money. You can pay me for some of the filing fees as you can. We will figure out what to do."

In the beginning, Santa Fe totally refused to hold the hearing in Las Cruces. I was supposed to travel there, 290 miles, but I had women with babies due and no backup. Stephanie was able to force the State of New Mexico into changing the venue to Las Cruces where the incident happened.

There was a lot of paperwork back and forth between me and Santa Fe about Bruder's complaint and my license revocation hearing. I had 30 days to prove my innocence.

The hearing was finally held on October 26th [1982] at the Las Cruces Health Department. Over a hundred people attended the hearing—my former and current patients and their mothers, cousins, migrant farm workers. The Health Department had no more room to seat them, so they spilled out into the halls.

Stephanie said that the problem was not that I had done anything wrong, but rather the way the regulations were written. I could pay for the indigent women to have their lab tests done and see the doctor out of my own pocket, but I could not see them for free for prenatal care. It had to do with some small way the regulations were worded.

My disclaimer form, stating that these women who had no resources to obtain labs and see physicians were not my patients because I was not going to deliver them, could not stand up to the test of this one clause in the practice act. Stephanie explained that was what they were using to nail me. They were revoking my license on this technical point of interpretation.

My case went public—newspapers, interviews on the ra-

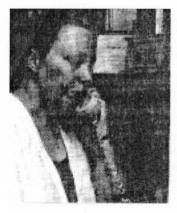
Photo El Paso Times

dio and on television. My picture was on the front of the newspaper several times. They used the same picture of me on the phone all the time. I guess this was a stock photo. It actually made the papers in Arizona and El Paso, Texas.

The State of New Mexico had two or three lawyers working on this. The State had depositions proving that I had seen a lady who was 43 weeks pregnant with pre-clampsia. And that I was not allowed to see anyone with pre-clampsia. Yet, I had thorough records to document that this woman had not been in to see me for two or three weeks. When she came to see me, I immediately sent her to the emergency room.

The hearing began October 26, 1982 and was over the next day. Stephanie had about 20 people ready to speak on my behalf. They had submitted written statements. After hearing the testimony of the state's case, Stephanie called only me to testify. It is all kind of a blur in my memory. Here is what the newspapers had to say.

Las Cruces Sun-News   Tues, Oct. 26, 1982   State/Local

Hearing Opens On Midwife Fate

By BRUCE HOLTGREN – Of The Sun-News

Dona Ana County's only licensed midwife may lose that license because she has allegedly been providing free pre-natal care to expecting mothers who cannot afford it.

A hearing was underway at press time today to determine whether Judy Lee, licensed by the state as a provisional registered lay midwife, will have that license suspended.

About three dozen supporters of Ms. Lee, many with infants and toddlers, crowded into the small hearing room at the Las Cruces field office of the state health department to hear the proceedings.

At the hearing, the state was attempting to prove that Ms. Lee provided free prenatal care to a pregnant woman in July. Counsel for Ms. Lee had not begun the midwife's side of the case at press time.

Ms. Lee's license was suspended Sept 9 upon recommendation from Linda Lonsdale, head of the health department's maternal health section. But Ms. Lee obtained a stay of that suspension, allowing her to continue practicing midwifery until today's hearing.

The state occupational licensing bureau suspended Ms. Lee's license after Ms. Lonsdale received a complaint from a Las Cruces obstetrician.

Under state regulations, a pregnant woman may not receive a midwife's care unless a physician first examines the woman and determines that the pregnancy is not a high risk. Once under the care of the midwife, the expectant mother is required to see a physician again between the 36th and 40th weeks.

"It's not that I don't agree with the regulations. I can certainly understand the reasons for them," Ms. Lee said before the hearing. But she said that her license was suspended because the regulations were interpreted to mean that she cannot provide care to women who cannot afford the physician's examinations.

She does not agree with that interpretation, saying it is "not in the best interests of the health and well being of the mothers and their babies. Some kind of prenatal care is better than no care at all."

Ms. Lee emphasized that she has not made any deliveries involving mothers who have not been given a physician's OK to have a midwife do the delivery. And she said there has been "no misunderstanding between the mothers and me" and that she has not been accused of "hurting anyone.

I have always given free care to anyone who cannot afford it and who asks for it," she said. "I've been doing it from the beginning, and I've made no effort to hide it."

She said she provides the free prenatal care because there is no other place in the county that such care is available, including the local field office of the state health department.

She added that the number of walk-in maternity cases at the hospital is "just enormous" and that many of those mothers have received little or no prenatal care all because of the lack of facility for free care.

The El Paso Times   Wed Oct. 27, 1982   New Mexico

Cruces Midwife Claims Doctors Refused Patients

By JOAN MORRIS

LAS CRUCES—A Dona Ana County registered lay midwife may have her license suspended if the state Health and Environment Department secretary finds she violated state regulations by providing prenatal care to women in the county.

Tuesday's emotional hearing on the suspension of Judy Lee was conducted by Health and Environment Division Hearing Official Tom Shinas. Shinas will make a recommendation to the secretary of the department.

Ms. Lee, the only registered midwife in Dona Ana County was reprimanded Sept 9 and her license suspended for the rest of the year on a complaint from a local obstetrician. The suspension has been stayed until her case is decided.

The complaint alleged Ms. Lee was providing free prenatal care to a woman who was admitted to Memorial General Hospital with pregnancy complications. Linda Lonsdale, head of the maternal health section of the department, said lay midwives are not permitted to give any care or treatment to pregnant women unless they meet the criteria for having a midwife-assisted birth.

Those regulations require all women considering home birth with a midwife to have two examinations by a physician and a series of laboratory tests. The second doctor's examination must take place before the woman enters her 36th week of pregnancy.

Many of the 40 attending the hearing were women with infants. Almost the entire audience, which spilled out into a hallway, was there supporting Ms. Lee. Ms. Lee who has been at odds with local doctors about her practice, admitted she had given prenatal care to the woman, as well as other women in the county. But Ms. Lee said she never delivered the women's babies or led the women to believe she could deliver the babies.

Ms. Lee also said Ms. Lonsdale was aware of her practice and had condoned and encouraged her to continue. Ms. Lee said one of the reasons she was giving prenatal care to the women was because local doctors had refused them treatment.

In August 1981, Las Cruces obstetricians adopted a policy not to provide examinations to women who were planning home deliveries. The doctors said if they provided the required two examinations, they would be condoning midwifery. The doctors said they opposed such deliveries as unsafe for the mother and child.

Ms. Lee said many of her patients were turned down by the doctors. Others could not afford the laboratory tests. Ms. Lee said if women told doctors they had no insurance coverage, they were told they must pay between $200 and $400 for the first visit.

A call to several obstetricians' offices in Las Cruces, made by *The El Paso Times,* revealed that doctors are charging up to $400 for the first visit if no insurance is available.

Dr. Murray Bruder, a Las Cruces obstetrician, made the complaint to Ms. Lonsdale. Bruder did not testify at Tuesday's hearing and could not be reached for comment at his office or home.

Ms. Lee testified Tuesday she had talked several times with Ms. Lonsdale about the problems she and her patients have with local doctors. Ms. Lee said Ms. Lonsdale, a registered nurse trained as a nurse midwife, knew she was providing the prenatal care free of charge to several women. Ms. Lonsdale denied any knowledge of Ms. Lee's actions. Ms. Lonsdale testified Tuesday that she had never condoned breaking the regulations.

Ms. Lee testified that in the past she has paid for the lab tests herself. But Ms. Lee said she stopped the practice because it became too expensive. Ms. Lee said there is no place for women in Dona Ana County to go to receive free prenatal care. She said many of her clients are poor, cannot afford the tests and have no transportation to El Paso or Alamogordo to visit doctors who will conduct the required examinations.

The complaint against Ms. Lee centers around Martha Ochoa, who allegedly was denied care by local doctors. The woman also was indigent, Ms. Lee and Ms. Lonsdale testified. Ms. Ochoa reportedly was in her 43rd week when she was sent to Memorial General Hospital in Las Cruces by Ms. Lee. A neighbor of the woman called Ms. Lee and told her Ms. Ochoa was ill. After Ms. Lee checked the woman, she sent her to the hospital. Ms. Lee sent to the hospital her report on Ms. Ochoa's progressing pregnancy. Ms. Ochoa underwent an emergency cesarean section and the baby was delivered.

Ms. Lonsdale, who denied Bruder or other doctors had put "undue pressure" on her to bring charges against Ms. Lee, said Bruder reported the incident to her and questioned whether Ms. Lee had disobeyed regulations.

Ms. Lee said she had cared for "high-risk" women, although she has not delivered any of their babies. "I would care for a high-risk patient if she had no place to go," Ms. Lee said. "I would provide prenatal care until or unless an obstetrical or medical problem resulted. If there was no other prenatal care available, I sincerely believe some prenatal care is better than none."

Cheryl Azarre of Las Cruces testified that she was a patient of Bruder but was "kicked out" after she fell behind on her payments. Ms. Azarre said she was paying Bruder in monthly installments for the examinations and eventual delivery of her child. Ms. Azarre said that when her husband lost his job, she could not make the payments. She said Bruder then demanded she pay the remainder of the bill immediately.

Shinas gave Ms. Lee and the state's lawyer until 5 p.m. Tuesday to submit final arguments. Persons wishing to give written statements also must submit their letters by that date. Shinas said he will have his recommendation prepared within five days of that date.

Las Cruces Sun-News   Wed   Oct. 27 1982

Midwife Presents Her Case

By BRUCE HOLTGREN

No decision has yet been reached on whether a Dona Ana County lay midwife will have her license suspended, but her side of the story was presented Tuesday afternoon at a state health department hearing.

Judy Lee, the county's only licensed midwife, said today that she does not expect the case to be resolved for at least 10 days to two weeks.

A Las Cruces obstetrician filed a complaint with the health department in July stating that Ms. Lee has provided free prenatal care to pregnant women who cannot afford to have a physician. State regulations specify that before any woman can be approved for a midwife's care, the woman must first be tested and examined by a physician.

Ms. Lee admits that she has provided the free care, but contends that she has done so with the knowledge of her supervisor, Linda Lonsdale, head of the maternal health section of the department. She also maintains that she must provide the free prenatal care because there is no other place in the county for such care to be found, and that she has never done a delivery without a physician's approval.

Ms. Lee obtained a stay of the suspension of her license, allowing her to continue practicing midwifery until the case is decided. After being delayed twice, the hearing took place at the Las Cruces field office of the health department on Tuesday. Attorneys for both sides were given five days to submit summary statements to the hearing examiner, Tom Chaines. Chaines then has five days to make a recommendation on the case to the secretary of the health and human services department, George Goldstein.

"I felt like I had the opportunity to explain that I was operating under a misconception," Ms. Lee said of the hearing. "I thought the hearing officer was very impartial in listening to both sides and in the way he admitted evidence."

Asked if she would appeal the health department's decision on the case should it be against her, Ms. Lee said she probably will not.

At the end of that first day of testimony Stephanie explained, "I think I can work out a deal with them. What would you be willing to do?"

This is a copy of the hearing officer's report to the State of New Mexico that outlines the deal that Stephanie arranged.

HEALTH AND ENVIRONMENT DEPARTMENT

Administrative Appeal

Health and Environment Department
Health Services Division,
    Appellant,

vs.

Judith Lee, Lay Midwife
Route 1, Box 221
La Mesa, New Mexico 88044

WITNESSES

Apellant
Respondent
Judith Lee

Linda Lonsdale, Head
Maternal Health Section, MSD

All testimony under oath.

Counsel for the State: Jerry Dickinson, Esquire
Counsel For Ms. Lee: Ms. Stephanie Blank, Esquire
Ms. Michell Olszta, Esquire

Findings of Fact:

Ms. Lonsdale testified that she had received a complaint that Ms. Lee had accepted in prenatal care, a client who did not have a physician's examination or lab workup as required by regulation. (Exhibit 6)

A letter dated August 18, 1982 from Ms. Lee to Ms. Lonsdale (Exhibit 3) indicated that she had provided prenatal care to women who did not have a physician's workup or lab tests. Ms. Londale testified that the patient, Mrs. Ochoa, was sent to Memorial Hospital in Las Cruces, New Mexico in her 43rd week with complications (Exhibit 4).

Ms. Lonsdale also testified that she orally discussed the subject of prenatal care regulation requirements with Ms. Lee at an earlier date. Because of the complaint and Ms. Lee's admissions in Exhibit 3, Ms. Lonsdale felt there was sufficient evidence to suspend Ms. Lee's permit.

Ms. Lee testified that she has been licensed since October, 1980. Her practice is located in the Anapra-Anthony area. She testified that she performs a great deal of free work, including occasionally paying for a physician's examination in El Paso, as well as lab work. Many of her clients are poor

81

with husbands out of work.

She testified that she did discuss verbally with Ms. Lonsdale at an earlier date (about February 1981) the question of pre-natal care. Ms. Lee testified she came away from the discussion thinking that as long as she didn't intend to deliver the mother, she was complying with the regulations.

She further testified that at the time she wrote Exhibit 3 she had another oral discussion with Ms. Lonsdale and understood the regulation concerning requirements under prenatal care.

Ms. Lee's intent not to deliver was also stated in her July 21, 1982 referral to the Memorial Hospital in Las Cruces, (Part of Exhibit 6) where she states the patient Mrs. Ochoa was pre-registered for admission at the hospital.

Recommendations

I don't believe the regulations meant to create a splitting of care. However, Judith Lee believed essentially that. Her belief allowed Ms. Ochoa to appear at the hospital in her 43rd week with some complications.

Had her interpretation been otherwise, she could not have provided any prenatal care at all to a woman who did not have the money to pay for a physician's initial exam, lab work or physician's visit in the 36th to 40th week.

I cannot condone Ms. Lee's actions, however well meaning and feel that her assuming the care of a patient requires all of Section 800 to apply. Her misunderstanding of prenatal care and plan to deliver and subsequent correction of the misunderstanding does not warrant the suspending of her permit for 106 days.

I recommend that the period of suspension be reduced from

106 days to 22 days commencing December 9, 1982, and ending December 31, 1982. If Ms. Lee attends the HSD-sponsored educational sessions for lay midwives in Albuquerque on December 9 and 10, 1982 (agenda attached) and attendance is verified to the Occupational Licensing Bureau, the suspension shall be lifted and have no further force and effect.

Thomas J. Shinas, Hearing Officer

I was already scheduled to attend the conference in Albuquerque. I had arranged several months earlier to have this time off and had a midwife who would cover my practice while I was away.

After the hearing was over, I continued my practice. Everytime I would have any kind of transport for whatever reason, no matter how exhausted I was the next day, I would take a basket of goodies to the nurses. Along with cheese, fruit and other things, I would tuck in a thank-you note. The labor and

_____ The nurses would take me

u. We are not allowed

ɔm the doctors about

complaining of some

woman— very young.

al, but you would defi-

1at was needed was an

was located and make

low lying placenta.

ɪ not accompany her to the hospital for the ultrasound for placental location. The hospital emergency room refused to see her. The husband and the wife called to tell me that they were refused services at the hospital. "Well, put them on the phone," I said. "I want to talk to whoever is there."

The ER person said, "We've been told not to send any of these women up to the labor and delivery unit anymore. You can't be sending people here saying that they need tests."

I asked, "If this woman walked in as far pregnant as she is and said she was bleeding, what would you do with her?"

"We would send her up to Labor and Delivery."

"Well, then get her on a cart and send her up to L&D. Do you want to take a chance and maybe have her bleed to death on the way there? We need to find out where the placenta is. She needs to be in the hospital to find out what is going on."

The couple called me back sobbing. The ER staff sent them to Labor &Delivery department and they refused to see them there.

"This is crazy. Where are you?" I asked. They were a block from the hospital calling from a store. "I am with a lady in labor and can't leave, but stay there," I responded. "I am going to call some people to come to the hospital and give you some help."

I got on the phone and called the lady whose dad was a lawyer. I informed her of the circumstances and asked if she could go to the hospital to help the young couple. Before leaving for the hospital, she called every pregnant woman that she knew from classes. They then called other women.

Within an hour and a half, there was a group of women picketing the hospital. They had little babies and buggies and kids around, and big handmade cardboard signs. They had painted messages like: **UNFAIR TO MIDWIFE - WOMAN COULD BLEED TO DEATH - CARE REFUSED.**

No kidding! They were there. The newspaper picked it up. I was at a birth and did not know what was going on. Once the picketing started, the hospital did see her.

I did not know the women were going to picket. I just thought the hospital would have 20 women in their waiting room and they would have to deal with them. I felt that would just cause some small ruckus so this woman could get the medical attention she needed.

I was unaware of this article appearing in the *El Paso Times*. It certainly demonstrates that the temperament was set for public demonstrations. The refusal by the hospital to give care to this couple furnished the trigger.

The El Paso Times   Sun Nov. 21, 1982   New Mexico
Edition

LC Women Rally To Aid Of Midwife

By JOAN MORRIS, Times staff writer

LAS CRUCES—A group of Dona Ana County women have joined forces to protest what they say is discrimination by some Las Cruces doctors who are refusing treatment to women who plan home deliveries with a midwife. Kate Goldsmith, the unofficial leader of the group, said the women are concerned that pressure by the doctors will force midwife Judy Lee out of practice.

"We are concerned the doctors are discriminating against women who have chosen an alternate form of delivery," Ms. Goldsmith said. "We understand that legally they can refuse service. But we feel they are discriminating against us because we choose a midwife or have no money to pay bills."

The obstetricians in Las Cruces have refused to return phone calls or to comment on the claims of the women. But in August 1981, doctors contacted said they were refusing to see women who planned home births with a midwife. The doctors said they considered the practice "barbaric" and not in the best interest of the mother or child.

The feud between the obstetricians and Ms. Lee first surfaced in August 1981, when Ms. Lee accused the doctors of violating state and federal laws by refusing to provide prenatal care to some women.

According to state midwifery regulations a woman planning a home delivery with a midwife must have two examinations by a doctor before the midwife can deliver the baby. The first exam is given early in the pregnancy, along with a series of tests. The second exam must be taken before the woman enters her last month of pregnancy.

But only a few doctors in Las Cruces were perform-

85

ing the exams. Many women had to go to El Paso or Alamogordo for the examinations. Others could not afford to make the trips, Ms. Lee said.

The recent confrontation between Ms. Lee and doctors could result in the midwife losing her license for a time. Dr. Murray Bruder, a Las Cruces obstetrician, filed a complaint with the state midwifery licensing agency claiming Ms. Lee was providing prenatal care in violation of the state regulations.

In a hearing attended by many of Ms. Lee's supporters, evidence was presented that showed Ms. Lee had been giving free prenatal care to women who could not afford doctor's care or who had been turned down. Ms. Lee testified she did not know she was violating the state regulations. She said she told the women she could not deliver their babies unless they obtained the two examinations and lab tests.

But Ms. Lee said she felt obligated to provide the care that was being denied other places. When it came time for the women to deliver, Ms. Lee said, she took them to the hospital where the baby was delivered by the doctor on duty.

Sue Nix, 21, is pregnant with her third child. She still owes thousands of dollars in doctor bills for her second pregnancy. Ms. Nix said the doctors have refused her treatment because she cannot pay the bill and because she supports Ms. Lee.

Ms. Nix also is barred by state regulations from having Ms. Lee deliver her baby. Her second child was delivered after a doctor induced labor. After the baby was born, Ms. Nix said it was discovered the baby was only eight months along in development. As a result of the premature delivery, the baby underwent costly hospitalization and developed a series of complications.

Midwife regulations list as "high risk" any woman who had had a premature baby, prohibiting that woman from having a home-midwife attendant birth. Even without that problem, Ms. Nix said she cannot obtain the necessary tests and examinations so she could become Ms. Lee's client.

Ms. Nix said she has had no examinations to test the

development of the baby and no prenatal care. When the time comes to deliver her baby, Ms. Nix said she will be a "walk-in" at Memorial General Hospital in Las Cruces.

"I can't afford to go to El Paso or Alamogordo for treatment," Ms. Nix said. "My husband is a student and I stay home with my son. We get $240 a month plus food stamps." Ms. Nix said she had gone to a doctor and had gotten undressed for an examination, then was told to get dressed and 'get out of the office'. I just wish I could get the prenatal care," Ms. Nix said. "I'm very worried about that."

Ms. Goldsmith, whose husband also is a student at New Mexico State University, planned to have her baby in the hospital. She later changed her mind and began seeing Ms. Lee. When Ms. Goldsmith returned to the doctor for her second examination, she was given a note.

"This is to inform you, you no longer are a patient," the typed note read. "In the event that you should desire to reinstate your prenatal care thru this office, you will be required to pay half of the total fee for prenatal care and delivery, on your first return visit."

The current cost for prenatal care and delivery by all Las Cruces obstetricians is $729.75. Ms. Goldsmith said she felt the doctors were attempting to "punish her" for choosing a midwife over them, and by demanding the payment if she was to "darken their door".

Vickie Campbell, a Las Cruces woman who plans to become a midwife, said prenatal care is the most important aspect in pregnancy. She said the doctors are endangering the lives of mothers and unborn children by denying some women that care. "The doctors are refusing to accept the issues," Ms. Campbell said. "The issue is not whether midwives are good or bad. We have regulations to monitor them and license them. The state already has said there will be midwives in New Mexico. The real issue is that health care standards are being lowered when women cannot have prenatal care unless they choose to have a baby in a hospital," she said.

Ms. Campbell said she felt the doctors are denying

the rights of women to choose the way they want to have a baby. Ms. Goldsmith said, "No one has the right to tell me how I can have my baby. The doctors," Ms. Goldsmith said, "are saying you can either have the baby with me, or you can have it by yourself."

Ms. Lee said she is awaiting word on whether her license will be suspended. She said she has no idea what the decision will be, but in case her license is suspended, Ms. Lee has made arrangements for another midwife to handle her patients through January. Ms. Lee said she had planned to take a month vacation and already had arranged for the other midwife to fill in for her. "It's just fortunate she could make it now," Ms. Lee said.

Ms. Lee said her continuing battle with the doctors will not force her into another profession or city. "I'm going to be around for a long time," Ms. Lee said. "I'm not going down without a fight. I definitely plan on staying in business."

In the meantime, her supporters say they want to monitor the doctors' activities. Ms. Goldsmith said if the situation worsens, they will consider rallies, protests and pickets.

Other supporters of Ms. Lee are organizing a defense fund in case Ms. Lee's license is revoked, or in the event women want to file a federal civil suit against the doctors, formally charging denial of rights.

I had sent other indigent women into the hospital and viewed the treatment of this couple as the hospital's way of retaliation. They were trying to get back at me and they were using my women. They were putting the lives of my patients in danger to do so—vaginal politics at its worst! And they were using them to put me out of business by making it look like I was doing something unsafe.

The El Paso Times   Tuesday,   Nov. 23, 1982
New Mexico Roundup

Midwife Protest spreads

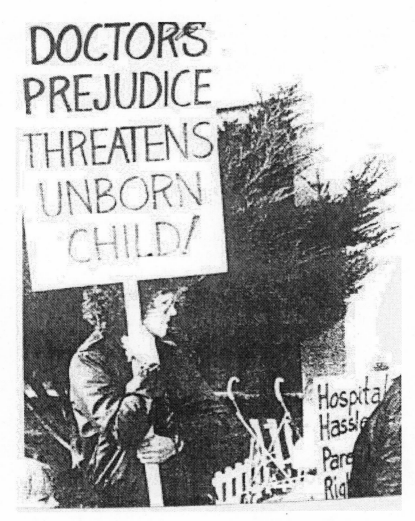

Tuesday November 23, 1982   Sun News photo by Bruce Holtgren

Angry Moms

Two of about a dozen mothers who demonstrated Monday in front of Memorial General Hospital talk about the situation. The women were protesting what they say are discriminatory policies by physicians who practice at MGH.

LAS CRUCES—About 20 protesters began picketing Memorial General Hospital Monday after a couple claimed that discrimination against midwives caused a bleeding pregnant woman to wait an hour before she was admitted to the hospital emergency room.

Hospital officials claimed there is no discrimination against women who want their babies delivered by a midwife. They claim the woman had to wait because she refused to see a doctor at the hospital until her midwife arrived.

Chris Jackovich said his wife, Sharon, who is past her eighth month of pregnancy, started bleeding early Monday morning. He said he called the midwife, Judy Lee, who told the couple to go to the hospital for an ultrasound scan to determine the cause of the bleeding.

Jackovich said that when the couple got to the hospital at about 8 a.m., they told someone working in the emergency room that the woman was bleeding and that Ms. Lee had said to get the ultrasound test. He said the woman refused to admit Mrs. Jackovich and did not offer to have a doctor examine her.

Ms. Jackovich's condition was unknown late Monday. Hospital spokesmen said the woman did not want to be interviewed. Ms. Lee said it is possible that Mrs. Jackovich suffered partial peeling of the placenta, which she said could be fatal to the woman and her baby.

Albuquerque Journal   November 24, 1982

Hospital Protest Overblown, Says Kin Of Patient

By ERIN SHAY – Of the Journal's Las Cruces Bureau

LAS CRUCES—Monday's picketing of Memorial General Hospital here was much ado about nothing, according to the mother-in-law of the pregnant woman on whose behalf the demonstration was held.

The picketing was organized after Chris Jackovich and midwife Judy Lee claimed that Jackovich's wife, Sharon, was refused service at the Memorial General Emergency room, something hospital officials denied. Ms. Jackovick who is 37 weeks pregnant, awakened Monday morning with heavy vaginal bleeding and went to the emergency room on the midwife's recommendation. Ms. Lee is a lay midwife, not a nurse-midwife.

Jackovich and Ms. Lee said Mrs. Jackovich was denied service for more than an hour and was not allowed to see a physician until Ms. Lee threatened emergency room employees with a lawsuit. Hospital officials on the other hand, contended Monday afternoon that Mrs. Jackovich declined to see a physician, preferring instead to wait outside the emergency room until her midwife arrived.

On Tuesday, Tully Jackovich, Chris Jackovich's mother, said the picketing and the presence of media personnel brought unnecessary attention to an otherwise ordinary incident. "You have to wait in any hospital," Tully Jackovich said. "They may run you up and down the hall a bunch of times and it seems like nobody cares about you, but that's just the way they work.

"They were scared," she said, referring to her son and wife. "It was a new experience for those kids. To my son that hour they waited seemed like a million years." Mrs. Jackovich said her son and daughter-in-law, who was released from the hospital Tuesday, chose not to talk to the media.

"It's all over; it's yesterday's news," Tully Jackovich said. "We need these people (at Memorial General) in our community. We were born and raised here, and we don't want to cause any trouble."

Kevin Andrews, administrator at Memorial General, agreed that an unusual amount of attention was focused on an otherwise not unusual situation. "As far as we were concerned, there was no fuss," Andrews said Tuesday. "When (Mrs. Jackovich) accepted a physician, she was given care. She was admitted as a patient of the hospital and has just been released."

Andrews said he thought the media have been manipulated as a result of recent hearings concerning whether the state will suspend Ms. Lee's license to practice midwifery. The hearing was held after the director of the maternal care division of the state Health and Environment Department charged Ms. Lee with giving free prenatal care to women not eligible under state regulations for a midwife's services.

Ms. Lee said Tuesday she learned unofficially that her license will be suspended from Dec. 9 through the end of December. She said she already had planned a vacation during that time. She will attend a midwifery workshop while another midwife takes care of Ms. Lee's clients.

In response to Andrew's accusation, Ms. Lee said she called in the media because she felt the public ought to know about what could have been a life-or-death situation for Mrs. Jackovich. "I wanted to make sure it didn't happen again," Ms. Lee said.

She said a lack of communication may have been responsible for the whole incident, but contended a breakdown in communication should not pose a threat to an emergency patient. "Anytime anyone presents herself at the hospital and says she is bleeding and they don't even offer to take a blood pressure, that's a miscommunication that's not in the best interest of the patient," Ms. Lee said. "If there were any miscommunications or errors, they should have been in the patient's favor."

Ms. Lee said she believes the hospital has refused service to patients in the past, though hospital officials say they routinely serve patients who are indigent or, like the Jackovishes, are uninsured.

Kate Goldsmith, organizer of Monday's picketing and leader of the group of women who said they want better maternal health care in Las Cruces, is attempting to compile statistics on patients who have not received services at the hospital, Ms. Lee said.

(Author's Note: The following interview with Laurete Francescato was part

of research for a different book. I had no prior knowledge she had had a home birth or that Judy Lee was the midwife who delivered her. Nor did I know that she participated in picketing Memorial Medical Center for Judy Lee.)

Laurete's Story (Formerly Mary Kay Fristoe)

My husband was not in the delivery room with my first birth. This first baby weighed nine pounds so it was a lot of work to deliver that child. I remember very little about it.

Before the birth of my second child, I did some reading, trying to educate myself. My husband was in the delivery room but that is about all I remember.

Now, here I am in New Mexico, years after having had a tubal ligation, with a new husband who wants children. I went through surgery having my tubes untied and got pregnant. Dr. Bruder was a popular person to go to. I saw him and Dr. Duarte, his partner, at the start of my pregnancy.

I don't know who introduced me to the concept of midwifery and home birth. Somewhere a friend must have said something to me. It sounded so delightful to be able to give birth at home, in home surroundings, have chocolate cake after the birth.

I started checking around and found Judy Lee's name. I went to talk to her. I was enamored with her gentleness and her love and her compassion and her nurturing. At that point I was still early in the pregnancy. I told Dr. Bruder I was thinking of having a home birth. He said that really was not a good idea, that midwives kill babies. I thought his response was pretty bizarre.

On a subsequent visit, I was seen by his partner, Dr. Duarte. He was very open to midwifery. He said his wife had had some problems with her pregnancy; otherwise, she would have given birth at home. He was supportive, but if I decided to give birth with the midwife, he could not be involved. You had to get some kind of approval from an MD on paper to give birth at home at that time. I ended up having to go to a physician in El Paso to get that permission.

I started prenatal care with Judy. I introduced my husband to the process of midwifery and home birth. He had never had children, so he did not have any experience with hospital births.

Judy asked her clients to sign an agreement concerning more than one woman in labor at the same time. If Judy was at a home with a laboring woman and another client started labor, the second woman in labor would be brought to the first woman's house so Judy could be present for both.

A week before I actually delivered I had an episode of hard contractions and called Judy to my home. While she was there another woman started labor and was brought to my house. By the time she arrived and was settled in with true labor, my contractions had stopped.

My children were not excited about the idea of home birth. Tammy was thirteen and Grady was eleven. They thought their hippie mother was doing something weird again.

So, this woman comes to our home and I get Tammy out of bed. She labors and gives birth in Tammy's bed. I was just so excited. It was a wonder to have someone giving birth at my house. To be able to run around and help and hear the sounds of labor. I was not concerned that my labor had stopped. It was wonderful to be blessed with a birth experience at our home, to have a baby born and watch Judy do her thing. And then see this wonderful little being enter the world.

I remember being so excited to be able to cook this woman breakfast and get her what she needed. A funny family thing, when Tammy had gotten out of her bed, she had gone to sleep in one of the twin beds in my younger son's room. She slept in one of his beds and ignored the whole birth thing. The next day or so she was talking about not being able to believe that, "My mother let somebody give birth in my bed." Then Grady pipes up and says, "What are you upset about? You started your period in my bed, that's really gross." Mother earth was just hovering over this house.

It was finally my turn a week later. I was ecstatic! Now I got to do the birthing thing. Everybody was saying things like, "You are over thirty-six years old. It has been thirteen years since you had a baby. Aren't you afraid to have a home birth?" The only thing I was afraid of was having to go to the hospital.

My previous babies were born sunny side up. (face up) Both of the labors had been long hours of work. I started in labor—it was just great, so fun—I was at home and I woke up at four in the morning. I swear this little boy was poking his fingers into the sides of the water bag. It felt like this baby was saying, "Okay, I'm coming out", and he was tearing the bag. This sounds absurd, but that is how it felt to me.

The water broke at five and I called Judy at six. She came to the house. It was really sweet. She stayed there with me the whole time. I could be up walking around in the house and into the garden. Then, I would hang out in my bed for a while. We spent a lot of time just talking, Judy and me.

Tammy was there and Grady was there. I don't know how they occupied themselves. I guess they were just in and out and about. I know that later Tammy mentioned that it was hard for her to hear me when I was into the hard labor and making a lot of noise.

I gave birth sitting in my bed. Norm, my husband, was supporting me from behind. At the actual birth event, Grady and Tammy came in and my friends Jackie and Robert were there. Robert was taking pictures. It was just a time of people coming and going and talking. There was no stress. It was a celebration day. Not having had a baby for thirteen years, it was an incredible place for me to be, having the opportunity to give birth and have this child come into my life.

Norm cut the cord. Grady and Tammy gave Josh his first bath. Then they wrapped him up and I nursed him and we had champagne and chocolate cake. I remember it was so neat, Judy showing me the placenta with all the roots and branches of vessels.

I was up in no time, taking a shower, and walking around outside in the garden. I had just given birth and I got to do all these things. I felt so energized and so charged up. I had no drugs. I had a great appetite right afterwards. It was an awesome experience.

Later, I had a problem with Bruder. He knew that I had given birth at home. I got pregnant again right away. I started bleeding with severe cramps. We kept calling him and he would not return the calls. I can't remember the conversations with his office staff, but the gist of it was he was not going to see me for this matter because I had given birth at home. At that point, my husband, who can be very vocal, called him and said that it was unethical to turn me down as a patient because of having a home birth. He agreed to see me. I went in and was told I was having a miscarriage. That is pretty much my dealing with Dr.

Bruder.

Later, I can't remember how the picketing got started or who started it. When I heard about it, my response was, "Of course, I will be a part of that."

We were hearing stories that things were getting hairy for Judy at the hospital. One of the doctors filled her shoes with water one time when she was in with a patient. They were doing punitive little things to her besides the big things.

My husband was an employee of the hospital in the Comptroller's office and I was out there carrying a sign. I remember someone bringing my husband to look out the window. People went into his office and asked him if he knew that his wife was outside picketing.

My husband was not upset that I was part of the picket line. There was so much political stuff going on against midwifery. He was supportive and was as upset with what was happening with midwifery at that time as I was. He did undergo some duress because everyone knew that I was his wife. He was certainly supportive of Judy Lee. He thought she was wonderful.

I do know that Bruder seemingly was on a real tirade to have her not practice any more. A lot of it just seemed to be so silly because he had a huge practice. Her business was not going to affect his finances whatever. It seemed like it was a vendetta.

Word got out among the indigent women that if the hospital staff knew you had been seen by the midwife you would be mistreated. They were coming back to me with their babies, talking about how terribly they were treated. The doctors were rude to them and would deliberately perform rough examinations. They reported being yelled at and told they would not have any of their problems if they had not gone to a midwife.

So the Hispanic community passed the word not to take any prenatal records to the hospital because they would get you in trouble. The hospital would treat you better if you had not been seen by the midwife. It was dreadful having women with records feeling like they could not show them at the hospital because they would receive abusive treatment from the doctors for coming to see me.

Drs. Bruder and Braden at the time were the head honchos. My challenging Braden on his drinking did not help.

A month later the official ruling come down from the State. The publicity said I was a bad girl. I got punished. They ruled I could not do any free prenatal care. My punishment was attending three days of continuing education in Albuquerque.

The El Paso Times Nov. 30, 1982   New Mexico Edition

Midwife Put On Suspension For 3 Weeks

Times Las Cruces Bureau
LAS CRUCES—A Las Cruces midwife charged with providing prenatal care in violation of state regulations has had her license suspended.

Judy Lee said her midwife license will be suspended from Dec. 9 through Dec. 31. She said her license will be renewed Jan. 1 if she attends a conference on midwifery in Albuquerque Dec. 9 and 10. Ms. Lee said she had planned to take a vacation for those three weeks before the decision was announced last week by George Goldstein, Director of the Health and Environment Division. She said she already had asked another midwife, Meg Harlam, to treat her clients during that time.

Ms. Lee said she was happy about the decision, since she was facing a possible three month suspension.

Murray Bruder, a Las Cruces obstetrician, filed the complaint alleging Ms. Lee was giving prenatal care to pregnant women.

At her hearing Oct. 26, witnesses said Ms. Lee was giving care to women who could not afford a doctor or who had been turned away by Las Cruces doctors.

Ms. Lee has claimed that Las Cruces obstetricians have been trying to sabotage her practice by refusing to see women who decide on a midwife-assisted birth. She also has claimed some obstetricians have given her clients drugs they didn't need.

Las Cruces obstetricians have refused to comment on her accusations.

Ms. Lee said the decision came as a relief and she will attend the conference in Albuquerque. "I thought it was a very compassionate decision," Ms. Lee said. "I think the hearing officer (Thomas Shinas of the Health and Environment Division) listened to what was being said."

The El Paso Times   Wednesday   Dec. 15. 1982

State Reinstates License For Las Cruces Midwife

By DOUG DesGEORGES

LAS CRUCES—A midwife who thought her license would be suspended for offering prenatal care to women too poor to pay a doctor said the suspension has been lifted.

Judy Lee said she learned the suspension was lifted because she had attended a workshop in Albuquerque for midwives.

Ms. Lee said she was told she would have her license suspended for 22 days beginning Dec. 9, the day the workshop started. She said she thought part of her suspension required her to attend the workshop, which she said she had planned to attend anyway. However, Ms. Lee said she learned that attending the workshop erased her suspension and she is free to resume her practice.

Dr. Murray Bruder, a Las Cruces obstetrician, charged Ms. Lee with providing prenatal care in July. She had a hearing on the charges in late October.

She said she received the final report from the hearing examiner, who said he thought it strange no doctors provide prenatal care for poor women. She said that is still the case and women who cannot afford that care still have to go to the hospital as walk-in patients.

Ms. Lee also said she has not heard from any local obstetricians since the hearing. "They don't contact me, they contact other people," she said.

State regulations require women using a midwife to visit a doctor twice, once early in pregnancy and once in the last month of pregnancy.

Ms. Lee said she now is taking a vacation she had planned before the hearing. If her suspension had not been lifted, it would have come during her vacation. She said licensed midwife, Meg Harlam, is taking care of her clients while she is vacationing.

This was a really good turning point for the community. There had been all this publicity about no indigent prenatal care. The university women and other middle class women were very vocal, questioning how we could have a health department that does not have prenatal care for poor women.

Within a month the health department hired Sister Angela, a Catholic nun and a Certified Nurse-Midwife, to furnish prenatal care in Anthony. I did not know her. I understand she was quite controversial and a powerful woman in her own right. When she came to the community and opened the clinic in Anthony, I called on her. I told her how thrilled I was at having her practicing in the community.

She greeted me warmly and told me that she had to keep a low profile. Her supervisor informed her that she had to distance herself from me and everything that I did. She could not help me or be part of my medical back up. It was nothing personal on Sister Angela's part.

After the hearing was over and I got that little slap on the wrist for what I had supposedly done wrong, I continued my practice. I stopped the free prenatal clinics. The community had some prenatal health care provided by Sr. Angela which targeted the indigent but things did not get better for me.

I was still having problems getting insurance companies to pay delivery claims in a timely manner. The women with insurance were paying me up front and having to wait for months to get reimbursed by their insurance companies. We decided we had to take action. Stephanie Blank offered to help us. The women from the university, along with Stephanie and me, did some brain storming and decided the best thing to do was to go to the state legislature and get the laws regarding insurance changed.

It was not just midwives who were having trouble getting reimbursements. Chiropractors were also having problems with insurance companies. Stephanie helped draft the actual legislation. The new wording read: any insurance company which does business in the state of New Mexico and offers coverage of any type in their policy will be required to pay any licensed provider who is willing to provide the service, if such service was a benefit of the insurance coverage plan.

We knew of several Democratic representatives and senators who would likely sponsor the legislation. Nevertheless, we felt our best strategy would be to gain the backing of conservative Republicans in the state. We asked around Dona Ana County and found Patricia Dominguez, a conservative Republican legislator. She was willing to meet with us and talk about the possibility of sponsoring the legislation. It turned out that she did not support home birth or out of hospital birth personally. Even though she had no vested interest, however, she did feel that any woman who paid insurance premiums should be able to use those benefits anywhere she chose.

She agreed to sponsor the legislation, HB 179, titled "Midwives Insurance". Now we had to develop our own tactics and educate the legislators and the public about home birth and midwives. We decided our best strategy would be to keep everything under wraps as much as possible until the pending legislative bills actually became public.

A person at the information center of the National Organization for Women guided us. We set up what we called a telephone tree for legislative action. This was composed of NM members of NOW, other feminists groups around the state, and the midwives.

I rallied the midwives. We gathered telephone numbers of our current and previous patients. They expanded the telephone tree to reach out to their family members and other members of the community who supported midwifery.

We were able to get this set up in a very short period of time. We were ready for the bill to be presented. Our ground swell covered the state, but the majority of supporters were in the southern part of the state.

We decided our sponsoring legislator needed to have the hand-in-hand presence of a midwife who could speak on behalf of the bill. We midwives flooded into Santa Fe and took turns accompanying her all the time—in the State House, in and out of sessions, even going to the restroom. When she was questioned about the bill, she had an expert at her elbow to help with answers. This expert assistance enabled her to explain the safety and freedom of choice issues immediately and with authority.

It was well documented that home birth and out-of hospital birth in a normal pregnancy were safer than in-hospital for both the baby and the mother. Also, infection rates are significantly lower. We armed ourselves with documentation of safety statistics surrounding home births. We put this data into very simple language and prepared one-page handouts that we gave to each legislator as we talked to them.

Anyone who has been active in the legislative process knows that a bill gets put into committee where it can be shelved. So the more committees it is assigned to the more likely it is to be tabled, which in effect kills the bill. Most bills would go through one committee, perhaps two.

Our bill was assigned to several including the Conservation Committee. We could not figure out why in the world we were in the Conservation Committee because we did not know what midwifery or home birth was conserving.

We used our telephone trees to contact the chairperson

of each committee. Calls were made from all over the state in support of the bill as a freedom of choice issue. We passed through every committee.

We felt very strongly that we wanted this law, not only for midwifery, but for other willing alternative medical providers. Because there was such a short period of time to work on this, we did not have a chance to obtain support from the chiropractors or other professional groups. It was midwives, women and families supporting the bill and the freedom of choice it assured.

The medical association in the state did not originally oppose the bill. However, once the pending bills were published, they quickly rallied the state organization of nurses to oppose the bill. When we were in the Conservation Committee, several nurses appeared and spoke against the bill. We were able to refute all of their objections with solid statistics.

Afterwards, I spoke to one of the nurses who was opposing the bill. She told me directly the doctors strong-armed them into speaking against us.

The bill got to the floor of the house and the senate and was passed by a large margin. We were so excited. It was our first attempt at using the legislative process. The positive action significantly empowered us.

It was 1985 and New Mexico was the first state in the nation to pass this kind of legislation requiring all insurance companies that do business in the state to pay any willing provider. Since that time, 25 other states have used it as a model and passed similar bills. Today, is it called the "any-willing-provider" law. [1]

We started submitting the insurance claims for services rendered by midwives with a copy of this legislation and were getting reimbursed in a much more timely manner.

---

1. April 2003, a landmark decision of the Supreme Court ruled in favor of the "Any-Willing-Provider Laws" (currently existing in 25 states) to curtail rampant HMO abuses. Epstein Becker & Green, PC.

This empowerment gave us the courage to go forward with some other issues like of restraint of trade. I did not know for sure what the phrase implied. I knew that the doctors were doing things to make sure women having babies did not have freedom of choice. It was Attorney Hubert who defined the situation as restraint of trade.

The Arizona attorneys used the local law offices of Martin, Cresswell & Hubert to begin building a case regarding restraint of trade. Consultations began with the local ACLU representative. The law firm began requesting copies of my patient's records from physicians within the area and advising them that their firm was representing pending litigation. I began obtaining letters from my clients documenting harassment.

To Whom It May Concern

My son was born at home in Las Cruces during May of 1982. My experiences with local doctors during my pregnancy were traumatic to say the least. New Mexico law requires two visits to a physician in a home birth situation. My first visit was to a Las Cruces doctor. During this visit I was subjected to verbal harassment and made to feel as though I was wrong for wanting a midwife at home. It was so bad that for the second visit, I chose to visit a physician in Albuquerque rather than <u>pay</u> to go through that kind of treatment again.
     Sincerely,
     DeLaina Cushing-Cruver

Judy Lee
Birthways, Las Cruces

Dear Judy,

     In late 1981 I had an initial interview with you and had the lab work done in relation to my fourth pregnancy.

Then it was necessary in conforming with New Mexico law to obtain a physician examination. My family practitioner, Dr. Thomas B. Pettit, refused to provide me with the needed examination. It was my common knowledge at this time that none of the OB-GYNs would provide the examination.

Consequently, I did not continue using your midwifery service, but rather chose to use The Maternity Center in El Paso, Texas, where the physician statements are not required by Texas statutes. I definitely felt, and continue to feel that the physicians in Dona Ana County are not allowing women alternatives in birthing but are doing everything in their (very considerable) power to deny the women of Dona Ana County their right to choose midwifery.

I continue to believe both personally and professionally that women and families should be allowed to have alternatives. In March I will be presenting a paper to the Midwest Regional NCFR Conference in Des Moines entitled, "An Alternative to the High Cost of Birthing".

If I can be of any further assistance please feel free to contact me.

Sincerely,
Dr. Kathleen Eastman
Department of Sociology and Anthropology
New Mexico State University

Dear Judy,

When deciding where to begin my home birth practice, I did indeed hesitate to consider Las Cruces. I worked with Judy Lee for approximately one month in 1981 and soon felt the area OB's negative attitude towards midwives, particularly after transporting a woman to the local hospital.

The very hostile reception by the hospital OB's and the difficulty in getting the required physician consultations have been factors in my decision to practice in Texas even though I have been fully licensed in New Mexico for almost two years.

Cindi Cushing, Licensed Midwife

Dear Judy,

Norm and I really resent what is going on in Dona Ana County with regards to birthing choices. Having had the privilege of two wonderful home births we will do anything to help keep that option available to other expectant families.

I have had three hospital births, and there is no comparison to the wonder of a home birth. We treasure every memory of it. The midwife care pre- and postpartally was far superior to any physician care that I have received.

We feel it is totally unfair for any group of doctors to dictate what another doctor may or may not do. These harassment tactics do nothing to further quality care in Las Cruces. It simply forces more people to go to El Paso for services.

Mary Kay & Norm Fristoe

On behalf of the women in the area who had been denied "freedom of choice", we expanded the civil lawsuit to include "antitrust class action" along with "restraint of trade". I was busy working with my wonderful supportive women—delivering their babies and keeping them informed. The covert harassment had ceased.

I was planning to go to Chicago for three weeks, leaving my practice in the hands of one of my midwife colleagues. I was taking a much needed vacation with my family and friends. The week before I was to leave, I took it upon myself to personally visit every physician in Las Cruces who had ever refused to co-operate with their patients (or me) to furnish the state-required examinations and lab procedures for home birth.

My visit was short and my message was straight-forward and candid. I reminded them of the fact that their malpractice insurance would not cover any losses they might incur as a re-sult of defending themselves in a class action antitrust and re-straint of trade lawsuit, and I left town.

I heard through the grapevine of supportive nurses clear to Chicago, that Dr. Bruder was getting a whole lot of flak from the doctors he had strong-armed into refusing services to my patients. They were especially upset that they were going to have to pay out of their pocket to defend themselves against an anti-trust and restraint of trade lawsuit that he had provoked.

(Authors Note: The following conversation with Dr. Bruder is Judy's best memory, twenty five years later, of the way the conversa-tion went at the time.)

When I returned to Las Cruces, I called him. His recep-tionist informed me that Dr. Bruder returned his calls after 3:00 p.m. I started to leave my message and identified myself as Judy Lee. She immediately changed her response, "Oh, he has been waiting for your call. Hang on just a minute."

Dr. Bruder picked up the phone. "Hi, Judy Lee!"

"Hello, Murray." Nobody called him Murray.

He kind of sputtered but continued. "I understand you are having some trouble with your patients finding a physician to do their exams," as though he did not know what was coming down.

"No, not so much so at the moment," I answered.

"Well, I want you to just send all your patients to me and I will do their exams and labs for them," he said.

"I don't have control over the women who come to me

as patients. I do have some influence with them, but they usually choose the physician for these services."

"Well, I would be willing to see all of them for you."

"Dr. Morton over in Anthony has been seeing them with no problems," I answered.

"If you tell the women to come to me, I will beat his price," he offered.

"By how much?" I asked.

"How about three dollars?"

"You will give me a contract to that effect?"

"A contract? What are you talking about?"

"I don't do business with a handshake, do you?" I asked.

"Okay, I'll send you a letter. Oh, by the way, what is Dr. Morton charging for the visit?"

"Fifteen dollars," I answered.

"Fifty dollars?"

"No, fifteen dollars," I repeated, knowing the going rate for this type of visit was indeed fifty dollars or more. Dr. Morton out of the goodness of his heart was charging these poor patients fifteen.

"And you will agree to do the exams for the other two midwives who are practicing in the county?"

"Okay, I can do that," he agreed.

We dropped the antitrust class action and the restraint of trade litigation.

For four years I had been struggling to secure a letigimate place for midwives as an option to hospital births. It was a long and difficult fight. In the end we were totally vindicated. That my harshest critic should finally come to me and agree to everything, even to the fees he would charge, was indeed my sweetest victory. But more than the personal satisfaction, was the fact that women in this part of the state now had a choice. For that I will always be proud.

Part II

The Beginning and The End

Judy Lee

Midwife student

I was living in Evanston, a small city north of Chicago. It was 1976 and I was 30 years old, divorced, with a child. In addition to selling real estate on the North Shore, I worked as the assistant to the Senior VP of Barton-Aschman, one of the largest and most prestigious engineering firms in the US. We were working with mayors all over the country doing community re-development, using federal block grant monies, renovating downtown business areas.

Even though I held a highly responsible position, making decent money, I always felt that those who worked at something they loved were really lucky. I certainly never saw myself as ever having that. I was good at my job but I did not find it particularly emotionally rewarding.

I was part of a women's study group in the far North side of Chicago, in Roget's Park and another in Evanston. These were self-help groups dealing with women's health issues. We were reading feminist literature: Susan Brownmiller's, *Against Our Will; Men, Women and Rape;* Betty Freidan's work, *Feminine Mystique; Fear of Flying* by Erica Jong; and Gloria Steinam's work. *Ruby Fruit Jungle,* a lesbian novel by Rita Mae Brown, was from that vintage. We read stuff from the early '70's, e.g. *Black Women in White America, A Documentary History,* by Gerda Lerner.
I was also taking self-defense classes, as were many other women living in large cities. We were moving beyond the male view of sexuality of screwing as many women as possible, to the female vision of the right to say no as readily and as strongly as saying yes. The Lesbian movement was still in its infancy. Among my friends, we were sometimes called upon to proudly say "I am a lesbian" in order to demonstrate support for our sisters, whether or not we really were lesbian.

Also, at this time I had a boyfriend. We were saving our money to move to Israel. It was his dream to live in a Kibbutz, and I was part of it because of him. But then I read an article in the Sunday *Chicago Tribune* about a woman assisting another in having a baby. That was the first time I saw the word "midwife".

Once I read the story, I experienced an immediate and emotional "knowing" that this was what I wanted to do for the rest of my life. I re-read the newspaper story. It explained that midwifery was a career path for nursing.

I wanted more information. I called the teaching hospital in Evanston. The closest midwifery program was on the East Coast at George Washington University. To qualify for this program, you had to have a four-year nursing degree. The two year midwifery program was for a master's degree.

This was disappointing information. I never wanted to be a nurse. I never ever wanted to take care of sick people. These were the days when opportunities for women were pretty much limited to being a nurse, secretary or teacher. I had broken some barriers getting into real estate on the South side of Chicago. There were no women in the first real estate office where I worked. When I joined George Cyrus Realtors, on the Northshore, even they had only one other licensed woman in sales.

I prayed and meditated but I absolutely could not see going to four years of nursing school. I was quite depressed. Here, I truly had found what would be meaningful service and work, yet I was not willing to go through the pre-requisites.

During this time, my whole family went to Michigan for a few days to attend the funeral of a relative. At the service I met an old childhood friend, Christmas Leubrie, the granddaughter of the man who had died. During some of the quiet time, we had a chance to sit and talk. She wanted to know what I was doing with my life.

I told her about discovering this incredible profession called midwifery. But I was facing giving up a dream before even starting. I confided how depressed I was because I could not see attending nursing school. She told me there was such a thing as direct entry midwifery education. This educational entry program did not require a nursing degree as pre-requisite. There was a school located in Seattle and one in El Paso, Texas. She promised that when she returned home, she would send me the information. It was providential that all this came about within a period of a few months.

In a short time I had in my hands information brochures listing tuition fees, curriculum and entry qualifications. The information showed the school in El Paso offering ten times more hands-on experience. It seemed to me to be more important than curriculum and course work alone. I immediately decided the hands-on experience was for me. I made the decision to enroll.

I had been saving money to move to Israel with Ira. When my decision was made to attend midwifery school in El Paso, I got two part-time jobs. In addition to my regular 40-hour a week job, I tended bar on the weekend; and, I took up nude modeling at the Chicago Art Institute.

I never told my family what I was doing. I modeled for life drawing classes. I would not model for a photography class. I did not want any nude pictures of me floating around out there. I figured if they could draw me well enough that you could tell it was me, that was art!

My son, Jay, was in third grade. While my ex-husband had never paid any child support, and rarely exercised his visitation rights even though we lived in the same town, there was nothing in my divorce decree that required me to notify the courts if I was moving out of state. For some stupid reason, I felt I needed to do so.

I called an attorney. He advised me to go to El Paso, open a bank account and put enough money in it to show that I could live for a year on that sum. I should enroll my son in school and make sure that I lived in a safe neighborhood and had child care arrangements. The court would be concerned about these issues. The attorney would set up a court date when I had this lined up. We would go to court and tell the judge what I was doing.

There were no midwifery schools in the Chicago area. The only options in the United States were the Seattle School and El Paso. I did not see it being any problem, nor did my attorney.

I went to El Paso for the interview. I negotiated a timetable. If accepted, I would enter the program in the fall and my son would start the new school year in Texas. Because I had a child, they agreed to waive the requirement of living at the birthing center.

I was accepted and set up all the things my attorney had advised. I found a fire-proof apartment complex. A nurse lived downstairs with her small children. She was not planning to return to nursing and was very happy about the idea of picking up some extra money baby sitting, even at weird hours. If I was called to a birth in the middle of the night, I would be able to drop Jay off right downstairs and go to the birth.

After I was accepted, I had a discussion with my boy-friend, Ira. Although we had been together for two years and had plans to move to Israel, we had never lived together. He did not have a career. He only worked odd jobs. I told him that, because of the school load, I would not have time to date. It was my opinion that he needed to make a commitment to me and to the relationship and move to El Paso with me. He informed me he would not be moving to El Paso.

I had agreed to go to Israel with him, but he would not come with me to El Paso, not even for the couple of intervening years it would take to get my education. I was heartbroken and devastated.

Ever since Jay had been old enough to attend school, I would take off work the entire summer. We would travel the country and camp for the two and half months' break. As usual, we traveled that summer and arrived back in Chicago the middle of August.

Now I had to settle the house lease and dispose of six rooms of furniture, including my plants. I packed our clothes and personal stuff into a tiny U-Haul trailer.

Three days before I was to leave for El Paso we went to court. When I arrived, I found that my policeman ex-husband had hired a well connected attorney. They say Chicago has the best judges money can buy. And they do. He had called in some favors.

Although he had not paid child support or exercised visitation, the judge would give custody to him unless I stayed in Chicago. If I were to leave the state, then my ex got custody.

I saw it as a power play to keep me under his control. That had been a big issue surrounding the marriage failure.

I knew he did not want to be even a part-time father, and he really did not want to have my son living with him. I decided that I could not give up my dream of being a midwife. I refused to succumb to his pressure. I had it in my head if I just went ahead with my plans, within a month he would be so frustrated at having to care for a child, he would gladly agree to Jay's return to my custody.

Even so, I was desolate. They took my son from the courtroom at the end of the hearing. I did not have a chance to say goodbye to him. The court sent someone over to my place to pick up his things, the television for his room, and his toys. I was so distraught, I almost fainted while taking them out of the U-Haul.

I simply could not stop crying or get my head clear to do anything. Thank goodness I had already sold my furniture, and had the U-Haul pretty much packed. I realized there was no way I could drive. I would be a safety hazard to myself and others on the road. At this point, Ira, seeing what a mess I was, volunteered to drive me to El Paso.

It was a three-day trip pulling a trailer. On the way, we stopped at a couple of places where he had friends. When we arrived in El Paso, some of the staff from the birthing center came over to the apartment to help us unload the trailer.

We had barely unloaded the trailer when the school called me for a birth. I left Ira at the apartment. I did not see him for another 24 hours.

We did the birth. Before I could go home, a baby that had been born in the hospital came to us with a strep infection. The parents could not afford to keep it in the hospital. The baby was lethargic with a poor sucking reflex. It needed tube feeding, and the mother's milk had not come in yet. We were running around collecting breast milk from all these other mothers who were donating it. In my first 24 hours as a student, I learned the tube feeding of an infant. Looking back, I have no memory of that first birth on the day of my arrival.

I was thrown into an incredible responsibility. I ended

up spending most of the time with the baby. The other midwives were in and out of the birthing center doing births. I grew amazingly attached to the baby. All these events occurred within 48 hours of arriving, leaving little room for sleep.

Then the baby died. I had lost my son. I had lost my boyfriend. And now I lost this baby. I was a wreck. I was not sure I was going to be able to stay in school. Ira stayed with me another week, supporting my efforts to pull my act together. Then he returned to Chicago.

Missing my son, I got a library card at the El Paso library and checked out children's books. Then I bought a small tape recorder. I could talk to Jay and read to him on the tape. This gave me a reason to go on and a way to be in touch with him.

(Author's note: Judy is talking and crying. The weeping grows worse as this part of the story unfolds.)

This snapped me out of my grief. I was attending school during the day, doing prenatal appointments in the afternoon and in the evening, co-teaching Lamaze classes. I was also on call for births seven days a week, 24 hours a day. I had planned on completing the program in two years so that I would have a less hectic pace. When I lost custody of my son, I asked the administration at the school if I could finish in one year.

Shari Daniels, the owner and operator of The Maternity Center, was the one who could make that decision. She reluctantly agreed to place me on the fast track, but emphatically warned me that I had keep up.

I carried the tape recorder around with me, telling Jay about the new stuff we had learned in class. Then I would describe driving across the border to Ciudad Juarez, Mexico, for a home visit to one of the new babies from the night before. I described where I had lunch. My goal was to stay upbeat on the recordings for him, making it fun stuff. Once a week I mailed the tapes to him. I waited to call on the weekends when it was cheaper. Each time I called, my ex-husband would tell me my son was not there.

For months and months I was never able to talk to him. I asked my ex if Jay had received my tapes. He always answered yes.

School was an intense program. Shari's way of running things was as demanding as a boot camp. But we learned. We were doing 35 births a month, primarily in the birthing center. We were making home visits, one and three days after the birth, then postpartum care for the next six weeks. The six weeks postpartum period included well baby checks, nutrition and lactation counseling.

Three students and the instructor were seeing approximately 200 women a week. One of the students, Linda Holland, was an RN who had seen combat in Vietnam. She said Vietnam was only slightly worse than what we were doing. The other student was Loretta Manriquez. She was the first female in her family to ever leave home without being married first. It was a highly controversial thing. She went through tremendous family resistance. They opposed her living in the birthing center as a midwife student.

We primarily served a Spanish population, people who were in the United States legally and people coming over just to have their babies. Our care was much better than they could get in Juarez. Also the baby would be a United States citizen with implied privileges for the parents of a US citizen.

It was a hot political issue. I certainly felt as a parent, I would have done whatever was necessary to give my child a better life.

I spoke no Spanish whatsoever when I arrived. I learned immediately. It was pretty much "Spanglish" being on the Tex-Mex border.

Thomason Hospital was the El Paso indigent care hospital. We took some of the burden off their staff. At Thomason many women would hang out in the parking lot until they were pushing. Then they would go into the hospital and just pop the baby out so they could get a birth certificate. The nurses and doctors were doing the deliveries in the emergency room. It was dangerous. The staff was unable to do blood pressures or baby heart tone checks before the birth. They frequently ended up with babies with problems.

Initially the staff at Thomason gave us a pretty good

117

reception when we would have a mother transported. We would always go with the moms and the staff allowed us to stay with them. Within a few months, things began to change. There were some political changes involving the hospital, creating some hassle for the doctors. We were not sure what was going on. We students began to see our relationship with the physicians deteriorate. Our reception at the hospital varied from doctor to doctor over the rest of the year.

Shari did a really nice thing for us at Christmas time. Instead of giving presents, she gave us each a fancy pair of socks. Tucked in each sock was a coupon book. In the book was a real treasure, a coupon that could be used for a night off call. However, the night off had to be negotiated based on work load.

Within a couple of months, Ira decided he could not live without me and he returned to El Paso. I had been so heartbroken over his lack of support, that I was not receptive or open to being with him. I refused to allow him to live with me but I decided that I was going to use my Christmas coupon. Three weeks in advance, I preplanned a camping trip in the desert with him—just to spend the night sleeping in the desert.

I had to go through a huge rigmarole getting everyone's agreement. Finally it was on the calendar. As it turned out, the night I was supposed to be off call, we had several births. Shari called me for a birth but I was not home. So I had my night in the desert and caught hell for it afterwards.

We were constantly sleep deprived. The work load was stressful and the lack of sleep just added to the chaos. I averaged three hours sleep a night. The rest of the time, we kept crazy hours. My apartment off campus provided a place for me to get away but for only short periods of time. I know the other students were envious but they were also kind about it.

Several months before completing the program, I awakened with a horrible doubled-over excruciating pain. I went to the emergency room at Providence Hospital, one of El Paso's private hospitals. One of their OB doctors examined me and admitted me to the hospital. Twenty four hours later I woke up to discover he was not going to release me. I was suffering from physical exhaustion as well as a cyst on the ovary.

He was telling me that I did not need antibiotics. What I needed was rest. I tried to explain why I could not stay in the hospital or be assigned bed rest at home. I asked to be allowed to go home. He said only if I could give him the names of the people who would bring meals to my home.

I called Shari. She advised me that if I really wanted to be a midwife, I would sign myself out now. I was so unsophisticated I did not realize you could sign yourself out of the hospital. Of course, I had to sign their "Leave Against Medical Advice" forms.

I went home. The next day Shari came over with some injectable antibiotics. Although medical intervention was against her principles, she needed my functioning body. Instead of staying in bed for a week, I ended up staying in bed one more day and returning to work.

The birth center was located in El Segundo Barrio. The birth center itself was an old bordello from the turn of the century located within walking distance of the Mexican border. You entered the two-story house and were abruptly greeted by a large staircase to the second floor. Each room had little metal numbers above the doors. In its heyday, the girls and the rooms were numbered. They had left the numbers above the doors. We thought it was an interesting situation—this was where a lot of babies got made and many years later, it was a place where hundreds of babies got delivered.

Birkenstock sandals were our identity badges around the neighborhood. There were so many women living in the house, our neighbors thought we were a group of lesbians.

The police and the fire department knew us well. We did not keep curtains on the second floor windows of the bathroom. Our house was up against another building where no one could really see through windows. One night I was taking a shower and spotted a peeping tom up on the roof. We called and asked the police to cruise by. They actually sent a helicopter, but they did not catch our intruder.

For a while we received obscene phone calls. One guy

was making the calls. This was totally upsetting Loretta, who had lived a sheltered life in her Hispanic culture. What this guy was saying and threatening to do upset me, also, the few times I answered. It was sexual, not physical harm, but it was pretty threatening.

Linda, the nurse who had worked in Vietnam, put herself in charge of answering the phone. She talked dirty right back to him. She would tell him what she wanted to do to him when he came over to do things to her. He stopped calling.

There were stories floating around that the house was haunted. We were the school's second class of students, but no one told us about the house being haunted. They did not want to freak us out.

One night I was alone in the house caring for a newborn. The other two students and Shari had left the house to attend a birth off the property. I was downstairs warming some breast milk for the next feeding, when I heard someone call my name. I thought Linda had returned. I walked back into the front hallway and yelled upstairs. Nobody answered. I ran upstairs and no one was there. I returned to the kitchen and continued my task. I thought I was nuts.

Before returning upstairs, I stopped in the bathroom and I heard it again. I came out. I was sure someone said "Judy." I shouted an answer and went back upstairs. I was not frightened. I was just confused.

When the others returned, I questioned them. Did anyone come back to the center and call me? That is when Shari explained they had experienced some hauntings in the birthing center. The former students who had lived in the building said it was a common happenstance.

There were ghostly women passing in the hallways. Female forms were seen coming down the stairs. Every now and then, a client would refer to "that lady in the other room." We would question them and when we would go check, there would be no one in the front room. We did not want to tell them the truth, so we would just say things like "she is all taken care of" then continue what we were doing.

Since I lived in my own place, I did not experience this

often. It was only when the house was quiet that these phenomena would occur.

The barrio was a rough neighborhood. One of our patients called one evening when I was on call. In Spanish, she said she was having problems and could not get to the birthing center. It was not enough bleeding to call the ambulance, but it was something I needed to see about to rule out postpartum hemorrhage.

I drove over to the area where she lived, right on the Mexican border of the barrio. I knew that she lived down an alley. There was no number on the street for her dwelling. It was a rear second or third floor apartment in one of the tenement type buildings. I pulled up on the street. It was after dark. There were ten or twelve cholos with rags around their heads on the street. I told them that I was looking for Senora so and so. They were saying things in Spanish to me like "You are crazy! What are you doing here? Are you nuts?" I told them I was the midwife for this lady. They knew her boyfriend and they knew where they lived.

They found a parking place for me down the block. Half the guys were assigned to stay and guard my car and the other half carried my bags and guided me through the gangways up the stairs. It was real spooky. They led me to the apartment, knocked on the door and waited for an answer. They said they would wait for me and take me back to the car.

The woman was fine. It was just a matter of checking a couple of things and waiting to observe how much she was actually bleeding. I was there for a couple of hours. They waited. The numbers had thinned, but they hung out on the back porch. They carried my bags and escorted me back to my car. The guys were waiting by my car guarding it so it did not get stripped.

It would have been harmful for the woman to have walked down the three flights of stairs to get to the birthing center. The gang members cautioned me over and over while protecting me, "Don't be coming over into this neighborhood like this. You could get hurt."

There was always evidence of gangs fights. We did not know who was doing what. From two or three blocks all around us they would throw eggs, dye, paint or paint balls at things. But our building and the midwives' cars were never messed with. They knew we were serving their community and their women.

When we had a birth in our main birthing room, the three students would be present, rotating the management of the birth. One student was in charge of doing the blood pressures, another in charge of dilation checks. This way we all got to perform the normal duties necessary for a birth. Shari might not come until the active part of the labor and the actual birth.

Once we had a patient laboring at the birthing center. After a normal labor, the baby did not spontaneously breathe. It was the first time I had seen a baby that had to be resuscitated. Shari, Linda and I took the little boy from the bed to the exam table where the hard surface provided a space where we could work on him. We rubbed him and flicked his feet—the gentle things—and then we started puffing in his mouth. He had a good heart beat, but was just not responding. He was blue. We are talking to the baby, asking him to come into its body. "We want you here. You are welcome. Come! Come!"

As we are working on her baby, we heard the mom say, "And his name shall be called Jacob." We immediately began to call him by his name. "Jacob, come on baby, Jacob. Jacob, come on." And then the baby started crying after we had called him into his body three times by his name Jacob.

After that he was fine and had no problems. We took him to his mom. He was all wrapped up in his blanket. We started encouraging the mother and baby in the bonding process, touching and caressing. The mom had been frightened watching us work on him. Then she asked in Spanish, "Why are you calling my baby Jacob?"

Then we realized the woman spoke only Spanish. We had heard the voice in English. We asked the midwife who was sitting on the bed with the mother what she heard. She said that all she heard was us begin calling this baby by a name. She did not hear the part about "he is called".

We looked at each other puzzled. We knew what we had heard. We explained to the mom why we started calling her baby Jacob. She decided that was a good reason to name the baby Jacob although she had not intended giving him a biblical name.

While my memory of the first birth I attended was all a blur, I will never forget my second birth. A few days after my arrival, we had a delivery scheduled. We knew the mother was having twins. The father wanted no part of being there for the delivery. When the twins were discovered, he decided his presence at the birth of two babies was too much.

It was Shari's policy to have two birthing teams for delivering twins. All the details were laid out perfectly. We practiced who and how each person would perform her role. She grilled us and drilled us. The first team would be in charge of monitoring all vitals on the mother for the delivery of the first baby. Then one of us would take charge of baby number one. The second student became part of team number two and would move in to assist with the deliver of the second child. Shari would lead each team, assisted by two students with each birth. It was really exciting to think of helping deliver twins so early in my training. I knew I had chosen the correct school to attend!

I was assigned to the first team. It was my job to take baby number one, make certain it was all right, then provide a human body to take advantage of the baby's immediate and early bonding needs. Its mother was going to be busy delivering the second baby. Dad had chosen to be a non-participant. And there was no grandmother or aunt or other relative available to help the baby with the bonding process. This is important because bonding behavior in the infant diminishes after the first hour of its life.[1] The mother and baby can bond later but it is more difficult and takes longer. We did not want that baby bonding to some bassinet like they were still doing in the hospitals in those days.

Like so many twin births, the first baby was breech. We did the delivery right at the end of the table so its own body weight would bring the head out to the base of the neck. We wrapped the body in a pre-warmed towel to make sure that no

---

1. Klaus, M.H., MD. *Maternal-Infant Bonding: The Impact of Early Separation or Loss on Family Development.* Mosby. Sept. 1976.

cold air stimulus would make him breathe before his head was delivered. We made sure he did not rotate to a face up position. Then Shari "tucked his chin down" by reaching in and putting her middle finger in his mouth. She somersaulted him right up onto the mom's lower abdomen. He came out easily with absolutely no pulling or twisting on him, *and* with no episiotomy needed.

He stared at us and looked around while we suctioned his nose and mouth. He began to whimper a tiny bit but did not cry. We held him so his mom could touch and see him for a second. Then we had him latch on to her nipple to stimulate the delivery of the second baby. Nipple stimulation works great for getting contractions going strong. As soon as he started to suckle, she had another good hard contraction. The second baby moved lower in the birth canal. Soon mom started having the urge to push again. That was my signal to take baby number one away.

I checked his heart tones and did the five minute APGAR scores (a measurement of wellness and vitality). I kept eye contact as I allowed him to suckle on my (freshly washed) breasts. We had checked all this out with the mom beforehand to make sure it was all right with her. He was so sweet and quiet. Gazing into his eyes was like being transported to a heavenly place that he still seemed to remember clearly. I was just floating along in sheer delight. I had been rocking and cooing and loving this first little one for well over an hour by the time Linda came and told me it was time to bring him back to his mom.

By now, the mom was showered and cleaned up with her hair combed and back in bed. As I watched, they brought the father in. He was very happy and sat down on the side of her bed. Loretta, who had been in charge of the second baby boy while the mom showered, brought Noel in and handed him to the mom. Mom had had time with Noel before her shower. Both parents cooed over him. I stood in the background with "my baby" watching. After a few minutes, Shari signaled me to bring over Joel.

I stood at the bedside letting the parents touch and admire him. Shari gave me a stern look and signaled with her head to hand the baby over to the mom. I hesitated. Then she said aloud, "Judy, put Joel into mom's other arm so she can hold them both."

I did so very reluctantly. As soon as I let go of him, I burst into tears and ran from the room. It was a horribly unprofessional reaction. I was terribly embarrassed. I locked myself in the first floor bathroom unable to control the flood of tears. Linda came and led me to the upstairs. Shari did not want the parents to hear me. By this time I was also vomiting from the emotions.

I could not stop the flood. I had lost Ira. I had lost my son, Jay. That first baby who was born in the hospital had died. And now I was losing this brand new baby. These events were all balled up together. I could not separate the losses in my own head, much less in my heart. I knew I was being totally ridiculous, yet I could not stop my muddled thoughts or the tears.

An hour later, Shari came upstairs to have a talk with me. I knew I was in for trouble. But Shari was very compassionate. She did not yell at me. She explained that reading about the bonding process and "performing it with a baby" were two totally different things. She urged me to remember this experience and to be certain, if at all possible, to have a family member do the bonding. Then she said I had done a good job and had given Joel what he needed. She sent me home to my apartment.

I drove home, still very upset. I stayed up all night writing poetry about how I felt. I used up a whole yellow legal pad trying to get my feelings into the right compartments of my mind and heart. By morning, I realized that I had placed Joel into the same mix of my losing Jay and Ira. I was exhausted. But I went back to school on time and my emotions were under control.

Linda and I did the one day home visit. I walked in and immediately went to Joel. Picking him up, I called him by name. Everyone looked startled and asked why I thought that was Joel and not Noel. I said, " Of course it is Joel, can't you tell the difference?" They were so certain I had the wrong baby they checked the name on the ankle bracelet. Sure enough, it was Joel.

Over the next three month postpartum period, every time

we saw them, the parents and the midwives played the same game with me. "Tell us which one is which?" they would say. I never mistook the twins.

Throughout my midwife career, I made certain to have another family member present at births in case the mom had problems and could not hold the baby and bond. I was very careful to never, ever allow myself to bond with another newborn. I knew my heart could not handle it.

Twenty-two years later I was on a plane heading to a consulting job when the flight attendant addressed a young man sitting across the aisle. It was a familiar last name. I could not help myself. When the flight attendant moved on, I turned to the young man and asked, "Is your first name by any chance Noel?" (I KNEW it was not Joel.) He said it was. I caught my breath and continued, "Do you by chance have an identical twin brother named Joel?" He said he did, and was shocked to find out that I had attended their birth. We laughed and laughed until I was again in tears. All his life he had heard about the redheaded midwife who loved his brother so much when he was first born, that she cried when she had to give him back. And he knew that I was the only one who could always tell them apart.

Midwifery school was about life and death. I had never worked so hard or been so challenged in my life. Always before I had been a "B" student because I did not care to study. I listened well in class but barely ever studied. I was much more interested in reading than doing homework. I never considered myself a good student.

Yet now these women were actually going to be counting on me to know my stuff. I really studied hard. I was a straight "A" student. I could answer any question upside down and backwards. Even so, a lot of questions arose for me. Shari ran the place like a drill sergeant. It was so incredibly, "Do as I say and keep going no matter what." If she could keep up this pace with kids, a husband, and us, we "Darn well better be able to keep up!"

The more I learned about midwifery and my personal responsibility for supervising labor and births, the more I questioned Shari's approach. She was an excellent educator, but I could see she was not always allowing the women to flow with the natural process of labor. She was manipulating the births and situations in ways that I judged inappropriate.

Part of Shari's motivation was to provide the students with different birthing experiences. She wanted us to see everything. I was learning about birthing babies, but I was also sifting and adapting the information to form my personal practice philosophy. Looking back, I realize that was part of my development as a midwife and Shari's intent as an educator.

Before enrollment, I had never seen a baby born. Yet I never had a second of doubt about my choice of careers. I knew that I would be able to learn everything I needed. I totally believed in my acquisition of skills. We were doing some pretty scary stuff. I just felt that I could learn it and that I would be better for the knowing. However, I could choose not to do some things in my own practice. Also, part of being a student was learning what was done at the hospital as opposed to what we would do about the same situation in the birthing center setting.

Lay midwife or direct entry midwife credentials were not sufficient to get a job in the hospital. Illinois licensing was only for nurse-midwives. I could not go back home to practice. I needed to decide if I wanted to enter private practice or stay in El Paso and take on a teaching job at the school.

I really did not want to work for Shari. A lot of the things that Shari and her students were doing at the birthing center, I did not want to do in my practice. We were delivering twins and triplets. The school had a reputation for delivering breech presentations (butt or feet first) vaginally. We had women coming from all over the country to have their babies with us if they were breech. In hospitals, it was standard medical procedure to deliver all breech presentations with Cesarean section. We had a lot of women of different religions. The Jehovah's Witness women came to us, because they were not going to have surgery no matter where they lived.

Breech is no big deal as long as you know the specific delivery maneuvers and how to apply them. Physicians had always delivered breeches vaginally until the medical schools stopped teaching this process, forcing medical practitioners to move to surgical delivery.

The more I learned, the stronger my opinion grew concerning what was an acceptable out-of-hospital birth model. I decided that I was grateful for having the experience, but I also knew that I would choose not to take certain kinds of high risk patients in my own practice. In developing my own protocols, I quite clearly decided I was not going to be delivering twins at home. I was not going to be doing breech deliveries that I could not turn using natural methods. If I was the boss, this was totally my option.

Upon graduation, I worked a little while with a former graduate of Shari's program. Her name was Kathy Stanwick. She has done thousands of births in the El Paso area over the years. Kathy had a client who was having twins and wanted an experienced midwife rather than a student to help with this delivery. I went to assist at the birth. The mother had x-rays done and we knew there were twins. At the delivery, we were astonished when a third baby was delivered. She actually had triplets.

The doctor who had looked at the x-ray before the delivery did not see the third baby. One twin must have been lying exactly in the same position behind the other one. We went back and looked at the x-ray with him. The only thing we could see was perhaps a shadow of a second coccyx. The doctor who had read the x-ray was shocked.

That experience cemented my decision. I wanted nice normal births, done at home or at my birthing center. I was not interested in doing at home what, in my opinion, should be done in a medical setting.

I was recruited by a doctor at the Mescalero Apache Indian Reservation up near Ruidoso, New Mexico. He asked me about the possibility of living on the reservation and doing births with him. I went to check it out. I found out about the alcoholism rate and the drug use of the women. I did not want to work with that kind of population. Yes, they needed services. But I did not want that to be my first practice experience.

I had an offer at Arcosanti, a little community near

Scottsdale, Arizona. It was a community designed by Paolo Solari, to have no traffic, and be ecologically sound and environmentally aware. They had a very small population living at the facility in 1978. I would have a place to live but the expected volume of work there would not support me. I would need to make money for my food and expenses.

I had in mind that I was going to return for my son. I would need gas money, car insurance and other things for living. The only option for making money in that area of Arizona was to go to Scottsdale. The wealthy women at that time had a big interest in having babies at home. But I did not want to serve wealthy women either.

It was a very strange decision for me. What I really wanted to do was serve the wonderful migrant Hispanic women I had cared for as a student. The best location for this was halfway between El Paso, Texas, and Las Cruces, New Mexico. Coming from Chicago, I had been involved with the arts, theater and music. Both El Paso and Las Cruces had universities, theaters and music. If I could find a rural community between the two where I could easily commute to cultural events, this would satisfy both me and my need to expose my son to the arts. I found Anthony, which straddled the Texas, New Mexico border.

Court Battle and Family Sacrifice

My highest priority after getting out of school was to regain custody of my son. I graduated from school in May. I had until August to get my birthing center set up because the court hearing was set for September in Chicago. I was working night and day putting up walls, running gas lines and painting, doing all the work myself.

Then I returned to Chicago. Over the phone I had made arrangements with my ex-husband that, as soon as I arrived, I would be able to pick up Jay at school and spend a couple of days with him. When I arrived at the Catholic school as we had agreed, the principal knew nothing about my planned arrival. The nuns knew nothing about it, either. They were not going to let me take him from school.

I insisted they call my ex-husband. They were un-able to get hold of him. I had just gotten off a Greyhound bus traveling all the way from El Paso. I was tired and anxious to see my son. I got into an argument with one of the nuns who was assigned to watch me as they tried to contact my ex. I have never been a violent person but I almost punched out a nun. Being a woman who attended tewlve years of Catholic schooling, I knew this was pretty bad behavior. But I was frazzled and at my wit's end.

I demanded they call the police. I wanted them there. When the police arrived, I explained the situation to them. My ex-husband was a policeman and he was supposed to have made arrangements for me to be able to get Jay out of school. I requested they call on their radios and find him. This was bullshit that the staff at his precinct could not find him. He was ducking me. It had been a year and I made it clear that I intended to see my son.

The officers finally got my ex on their radio and had him call the school on a phone line. By this time, the supervisor from the police department had arrived to deal with this irrational woman who was insisting on seeing her son. The police supervisor got on the phone with my ex and read him the riot act. His final words to him were to let this lady take her kid. The police sergeant then put the nun on the phone and she received his permission.

Jay was thrilled to see me. I found out his dad had not given him any of the tapes. He had hidden them from him. Jay thought I had abandoned him. He knew that I loved him but he was hurt. This was the start of our weekend together.

When Jay was little and ready for kindergarten, I had moved from a blue collar neighborhood on the Southside. I did not want him learning racial epithets and looking down on people. I had purposely chosen for him a very free schooling system. We moved to the other side of the city into a neighborhood that was well-integrated so he could attend this school. The community had public housing as well as people living in multimillion dollar homes. There were Asians, Chinese, and Blacks. That was part of the concept of Evanston.

It was an excellent school system. They had incredibly interesting open classroom situations. The kids would take their spelling module out of a box. They would study and pass that module. Then they were required to teach it to another child before they moved on to module number two. They worked on the floor, or lay down, or crawled under desks, whatever was comfortable for them to learn.

As he began to open up over the weekend, Jay told me his father did not allow him to have any kids at the house. Even when his dad was home he could not have friends there. All the curtains had to stay closed, even though they were on a second floor.

And school was equally rigid. The thing that upset Jay the most was in his classroom, the legs of the desk had to be directly behind the legs of the desk in front. It was the most important thing in the classroom. After coming from such a free structured school, he was having difficulty adjusting. Everybody had to learn the same page at the same time. He was reading way above the grade level, but he had to stay at the level of the other students.

Judy Lee

I thought about his description of the school for a bit and then explained to him that he was really lucky. He had experienced both school systems and both ways of learning. He preferred to learn the first way, but he was also gaining an ability to learn in a very structured setting. This in itself was going to be good for him. When he grew up and he was the boss in a business, he could decide if it was his preference to keep the legs of the desk straight or if his employees could crawl around on the floor.

This really cracked him up as he pictured big adults crawling around on the floor like little kids. He thought it was funny and it kind of relieved the tension. I kept trying to make it a personal preference rather than right and wrong.

I knew I had almost no chance of actually getting custody. I felt I had to do everything I could to help Jay cope in the little time I had with him before I had to return him to his dad Sunday night. We had a great weekend.

We went to court the next day. I was trying not to be negative, but I was depressed and nervous. I was pretty sure it was a useless process. My economic situation as a recent graduate, non-established midwife was not promising. But I had to try.

My son dressed in a little suit and tie was sitting with his father across the courtroom from me and my attorney. The judge said that since I was just out of school, I could not show support. I did not have any income. His father could support him much better, and my child did not need to go with me.

The judge was about to make his ruling in favor of my ex-husband again when my son stood up in court and said, "Your honor, I want to see you in chambers." There was dead silence in the courtroom.

The judge said, "Young man, you sit down now. I am in the middle of something."

Jay stood up again and said, "No, your honor. I want to see you in chambers. This is my life we are talking about." The judge told him again to sit down. My ex-husband was trying to make him sit down. He did sit. The judge continued about how it was in the best interest of the child. The father makes more

133

money and can provide adequately. Jay stood up a third time and said, "Your honor, I want to see you in chambers."

The judge called for a recess. My lawyer was looking at me for an explanation about what was going on. I did not have a clue. The two lawyers and my son went into chambers with the judge. Twenty minutes later they came out. My lawyer gave me this knowing look. Reversing himself, the judge ruled that I could have custody. Just like that, Jay was mine. I was totally elated.

My attorney took the two of us to lunch. Between the courtroom and arriving at the restaurant, my attorney asked me privately how I got to Jay. He wanted to know what I did to make him choose to leave his dad.

"I don't know what you mean. I did not talk to him about anything. What happened in there?"

Lee said, "I'm both your attorney and your cousin. You can tell me."

"I have no idea. What happened in chambers?"

"Judy, come on. You told him to do that."

"I did not tell him to do anything. I don't know what happened." He finally believed me. I speculated Jay had been watching a lot of Perry Mason. That was how he knew to say that he wanted to see the judge in chambers.

When they got into chambers, Jay told the judge that he had lived with his mom for all those years by himself. He loved me. He felt that was where he wanted to be. He explained to the judge that while his father bought him a lot of things, when he would come home from school with problems, he was not allowed to talk about them. If he cried, he was sent to his room. He was told to buck-up and be a man. He felt like that was not good. He really needed and wanted to be with his mom.

The judge responded with, "Your mom cannot support you and your father has more money."

Jay told him, "I thought that might be what you were going to say. So with all this money that my dad gives me, I have been putting it away. I have it hidden in three places, not in the house. It is hidden where nobody will find it. If you don't let me go back and live with my mom, I want to let you know that I intend to run away from home every chance I get. And that I am going to get the money, and I am going to get on buses and hitch-hike or whatever it takes to get to New Mexico. I have maps and I know where it is. It is really dangerous out there. If you don't let me go live with my mom, if anything happens to me it is going to be your fault." He had dreamed that up by himself!

After that the judge gave me custody right there in the courtroom. I took Jay with me immediately. He never got anything from his father's house—none of his toys or clothes.

In the restaurant, we saw that Jay's dad was having lunch there, also. Jay asked if he could go talk to him and I agreed. He went to his dad and they talked. Jay tried to hug him. His dad pushed him away. I heard him say, "You made your choice, now live with it!"

When we arrived home in New Mexico, Jay started writing letters to his dad. I did not ask to read the letters and he did not offer. He would call his father and leave messages on his answering machine at home. His father was not taking calls. And he would purposely call the police station when he knew that his dad would be working. The desk person always told him that his dad was not there.

After a couple of months of leaving messages and sending letters to both places, Jay asked me if I would read one of his letters and tell him what he was saying wrong to his dad. I read the letter.

It was so grown up. It was about how much he loved his dad and what fun they had going to the drag races. He ended the letter with how much he loved him and how much he was looking forward to spending Christmas with him.

It was time for them to start making arrangements for Christmas so that he could visit him. Jay sent him the dates of the Christmas holidays at school, asking him how that fit with his plans. Was it time to start looking at plane reservations?

He was really looking forward to seeing him. Christmas would be the start of their new life together and they could make plans for the summer. He ended the letter with love and "I can't wait to hear from you."

I assured Jay it was a wonderful letter and his dad probably needed some more time. His dad never ever responded. So
the letters Jay wrote began to be further and further apart until
he finally gave up.

Returning to live me after being in the environment provided by his dad, required some adjustments. They turned into
learning experiences for him. He had a problem that I had sunglasses on when we were walking down the street.

"Mom, you have your sunglasses on."

"So?" I replied.

"Nobody has their sunglasses on. It is not real sunny
now."

"What is your point?"

"Don't you feel funny that you have sunglasses on and
other people don't have on any?" he asked.

"I don't feel funny at all. It is a personal preference.
Some people prefer wearing sunglasses later in the day than others. If you feel funny or embarrassed that I have them on, I will
be glad to take them off."

He thought about it for a while then said, "It's okay to
leave them on, Mom."

Living with his dad, he was exposed to rigid right and
wrong. There was only black or white. Prior to living with his
dad, there had been a lot of gray. There were certain things that
he had to do for safety, but if he wanted to wear pink pants and
yellow socks and a purple shirt, that was fine with me as long as
they were clean. He was used to dressing himself in his own way.
He liked bright colors. Then suddenly, he was thrust into a
Catholic school with uniforms that had to be a certain way.

When he came to live in New Mexico, things were a lot
more casual. He grew up in the public school system of Southern New Mexico enjoying the Anglo-Hispanic culture. He also
had his own horse and enjoyed other country-kid life experiences.

Over the years his dad never made any overtures toward
reconciliation. Now that Jay is a grown man, he has chosen not
to attempt any kind of relationship either.

Twenty Five Years Later

Judy -*left her midwifery practice in New Mexico in late 1985 moving to Thousand Oaks, California, where she went on to attend the MBA program at California Lutheran University. Her thesis reflected her continued interest in her chosen profession. Titled "*Psychosynthesis Personality Typologies of Nurse Midwives and Direct-Entry Midwives," *her research was supported by Midwives of North America (MANA) and the American College of Nurse-Midwives (ACNM).*

In 1999 Judy passed the National Association of Registered Midwives exam (NARM). This national standard of education and certification as Certified Professional Midwife (CPM) developed by MANA did not exist at the time she was practicing.

She has been invited to testify before federal committees in Washington, DC. She is author of EZ-DC Coding and HIPAA Management and is a contributor to Mosby's 6th Edition of Current Issues in Nursing.

Judy teaches and does private business management consulting throughout the USA and Europe. She continues to work part-time on a nationwide lecture circuit for a Tennessee university providing Continuing Medical Education (CME) for physicians and nurses.

She lives on a small farm in southern New Mexico with her faithful golden lab, Beau, two cats, peacocks, chickens, enjoying the vistas of the Organ Mountains.

Murray Bruder -*retired from the practice of medicine and sells real estate in Las Cruces, New Mexico.*

Drs. Love and Duarte -*continue their practice of obstetrics, compassionately serving women of Las Cruces and Dona Ana County, New Mexico.*

Laurete -*(formerly Mary Kay Fristoe) learning she was adopted, located her mother in Brazil, South America. Upon discovering her Latin roots, she changed her name to Laurete Francescato. She recently discovered her Brazilian father. Visiting Brazil regularly, she has integrated her American family with her Brazilian heritage. She is a Massage Therapist currently practicing in Las Cruces, New Mexico.*

Stephanie Blank -*left the practice of law to become a mental health counselor. She died in the mid 1980's.*

Shari Daniels -*In a career that started over 30 years ago, Shari opened one of the first Direct Entry Midwifery Schools in the United States, The Maternity Center, in El Paso, TX. She has delivered over 11,000 beautiful, healthy babies and is the founder of the International School of Midwifery in Miami, Florida, where her Florida students also receive clinical experience and instruction in Kingston, Jamaica.*

The Maternity Center - *Shari closed The Maternity Center. In 1987, one of her former students, Deborah Kaley, founded Maternidad la Luz, in the same El Paso-Ciudad Juárez community. She continues to train women from all over the world to be midwives. Since 1987, 7,500 babies have been born at Maternidad la Luz and more than 400 midwives have been trained there. MLL is a licensed birth center and is a nationally accredited education program.*

Alan Masters (Judy's ex-husband's Chicago attorney) -*In March of 1982, his wife disappeared. Six months later her car was retrieved from a canal and her decomposed body was discovered in the trunk with two bullet holes in her skull. Revelations of a long and involved police cover-up made national headlines, and Masters, along with his co-conspirators, were convicted of conspiracy to commit murder. A book entitled <u>Shattered Hopes</u> and later, a made-for-TV movie, recounts the stormy marriage of this alleged Chicago area lawyer to the mob, known in his circle as "The Fixer". Masters is now dead.*

Jay -*graduated from Las Cruces High School and attended New Mexico State University and University of Texas, El Paso. He went on to become* *a radio disc jockey, sports reporter, and production director for Martin Re-cording Studios. He is presently the production director for a radio station in the San Antonio, Texas, area where he lives with his lovely wife, Roberta.*

New Mexico Midwifery *—There are presently 51 Licensed Midwives in New Mexico. Thirteen are actively practicing. There are 132 Certi-fied Nurse-Midwives, almost all are employed. New Mexico currently has more babies delivered by midwives than any other state in the nation.*

The Author

Bette Waters is a retired Certified Nurse-Midwife (CNM), a Sexual Assault Nurse Examiner (SANE) and owner of Bluwaters Press. She lives in Las Cruces, New Mexico, where she writes fiction, nonfiction, poetry, and publishes books.

ORDER FORM

BLUWATERS PRESS
P O BOX 878
Mesilla, NM 88046

Call   1- 888-541-5381 Toll Free   MC/Visa accepted

www.zianet.com/bwaters   **bwaters@zianet.com**

Circle Title of Books Ordering

$15.95	**Vaginal Politics A Midwife's Story**
$39.95	**Wayfarers A Spiritual Journey of Nicholas & Helena Roerich**
$18.95	**One Foot Away From A Million**
$18.95	**Massage During Pregnancy, 3rd Ed**
$16.95	**High Sea Passages**
$12.95	**My Daddy Brought Me Up To Be Good**

Name:_____

Address:_____

City:_____**State:**_____**Zip:**_____

Telephone:_____**email:**_____

Sales Tax: Please add 6.5% for purchases within New Mexico.

Shipping: Priority Mail USPS $4 one book plus $.75 each addi.

Payment: Check MO Credit Card
Name on Card_____

Number:_____**Expires**_____

Name on Card_____**Amount**_____

Printed in the United States
1393700002B/259-306